ADVANCING
KING'S
SYSTEMS
FRAMEWORK
AND
THEORY
OF
NURSING

ADVANCING KING'S SYSTEMS FRAMEWORK AND THEORY OF NURSING

Maureen A. Frey
Christina L. Sieloff
EDITORS

SAGE Publications
International Educational and Professional Publisher
Thousand Oaks   London   New Delhi

For information address:

SAGE Publications, Inc.
2455 Teller Road
Thousand Oaks, California 91320

SAGE Publications Ltd.
6 Bonhill Street
London EC2A 4PU
United Kingdom

SAGE Publications India Pvt. Ltd.
M-32 Market
Greater Kailash I
New Delhi 110 048 India

Printed in the United States of America

Library of Congress Cataloging-in-Publication Data

Main entry under title:

Advancing King's systems framework and theory of nursing / edited by
    Maureen A. Frey, Christina L. Sieloff.
        p. cm.
    Includes bibliographical references and index.
    ISBN 0-8039-5131-0 (c. : alk. paper). — ISBN 0-8039-5132-9 (p. :
alk. paper)
    1. Nursing models. 2. System theory. 3. Nursing—Philosophy.
I. Frey, Maureen A. II. Sieloff, Christina L. III. King, Imogene M.
    [DNLM: 1. Nursing Theory. 2. Nursing Process. 3. Philosphy,
Nursing. 4. Goals. 5. Systems Theory. WY 86 A2444 1995]
RT84.5.A385 1995
610.73'01—dc20
DNLM/DLC   95-758

This book is printed on acid-free paper.

95 96 97 98 99 10 9 8 7 6 5 4 3 2 1

Sage Production Editor: Diane S. Foster
Typesetter: Janelle LeMaster

This book is dedicated to Imogene King and other pioneers in nursing theory who are able to relinquish the extension of ideas and ideals to which they are very committed. Fortunately, there are people who are well qualified and equally dedicated to this work. We are honored to be so trusted by Dr. King and we return our respect and admiration for her many times over.

Contents

Part II: Advancing the Systems Framework

Part IV: Evaluation

Foreword

For nearly four decades, Imogene M. King has participated in the strong evolutionary movement to carve out the unique discipline of nursing. She is an internationally known scholar whose ideas have influenced nursing theory development worldwide. The editors of this book have invited prominent international authors to describe specific situations about their use of King's theory and framework in research, practice, and administration. Authors from the United States, Canada, Japan, and Sweden relate how King's nursing theory guides their research and practice with adults, children, and families. The authors clearly demonstrate a logical connection between theory, research, and practice, further specifying nursing's identify within the discipline. The broad scope of the work is concrete evidence that King's framework and theory are useful to nurses in various settings around the world.

The publication of such a text on the use of nursing theory in practice and research, like other works of its kind, is particularly critical now, framed against the backdrop of the great controversy over the emerging role of the nurse within the projected new health care system in the United States. At this juncture, it is essential that the unique theoretical foundation of nursing be made more explicit with clear examples from research and practice arenas. This work contributes to that explication in general and expands the extant knowledge related to King's framework and theory in particular. It is a comprehensive text that makes a significant contribution to the literature of the discipline. This work honors Imogene M. King as a pioneer in the development of nursing knowledge and is a tribute to her commitment to and participation in the advancement of nursing as a science and an art.

Rosemarie Rizzo Parse, RN, PhD, FAAN
Hunter College, City University of New York

Acknowledgments

This book would not have been possible without the personal and professional support of family, friends, and colleagues; the mentorship, friendship, and trust of Imogene King; and the assistance, organizational skill, and exquisite attention to detail provided by Dianne Bailey. They all have my heartfelt thanks.

Maureen A. Frey

I would like to thank Imogene King, who has been, and continues to be, a mentor in my continuing theoretical efforts. I would also like to recognize Dr. Marjorie Isenberg, who was instrumental in fostering my interest in nursing theory. Finally, I would like to thank Mildred, Louis, and Doris Sieloff for past and current support.

Christina L. Sieloff

PART I

BUILDING NURSING SCIENCE

— 1 —

From Conceptual Frameworks to Nursing Knowledge

MAUREEN A. FREY

As knowledge development in nursing moves into the 21st century, its past provides clear direction for work to be done in the 1990s. The history, successes, and shortcomings of nursing are well documented in the literature (e.g., Fawcett, 1983; Meleis, 1991; Nicoll, 1992). Despite divergence, there is agreement in several areas. First and foremost is that nursing, as a profession, is responsible for its scientific basis, which documents its distinctiveness and separateness from, as well as interrelatedness with, other disciplines. Inherent in describing nursing as a science is that nursing should have an identifiable theory base. Indeed, nursing takes the goal of theory development seriously.

Basic questions related to the how and why of theory development dominated theoretical discussions and publications during the 1960s and 1970s. The 1980s reflected sophistication and expansion of theoretical, philosophical, and scientific thought and method. This included recognition of multiple approaches to developing theory, a second area of agreement. Also during the 1980s, attention turned to the many processes that contribute to furthering nursing knowledge: extension, examination, and evaluation of theoretical structures in research and in practice.

One path to theory development is by way of nursing's extant conceptual frameworks.[1] Conceptual frameworks are, by definition, broad but distinct views of the discipline of nursing. Conceptual frameworks have been likened to maps (Visintainer, 1986), lenses, knots (concepts) and strings (principles) (Hempel, 1952), and private images (Reilly, 1975). Each (a) provides a perspective of the metaparadigm concepts of person, health, and environment; (b) identifies other relevant concepts for nursing (i.e., adaptation, transaction, four dimensionality, self-care, languaging); (c) identifies relationships between concepts; and (d) suggests some focus and rationale for the activities of practitioners.

Conceptualizations of nursing are as old as the discipline itself, the first being traced to Florence Nightingale. Unfortunately, conceptualizations as approaches to nursing were not recognized or formalized for almost 100 years (Fawcett, 1989). Since the 1960s, the contribution and role of conceptual frameworks in the development of nursing knowledge has been a consistent theme in the literature. Although not universally agreed on, conceptual frameworks were to provide clear and relevant guidelines for development of nursing theory. Theory developed from conceptual frameworks was theory unique to the discipline of nursing. Practice guided by a nursing conceptual framework distinguished nursing from other disciplines, not only by identifying specific problems that nursing could diagnose but by identifying the ways and means to treat those problems (Fawcett, 1989; Fitzpatrick & Whall, 1989a; Huch, 1988; Phillips, 1988; Smith, 1992).

Several trends in the writings about conceptual frameworks dominated the 1980s: analysis, evaluation, and validity. However, the close relationships between these areas were not always evident because work was done by different persons, for different purposes, and not synthesized in the literature. Analysis and evaluation are probably the better known of the trends, perhaps because of the excellent texts by Fitzpatrick and Whall (1983, 1989a), Fawcett (1984, 1989), Parse (1987), and Meleis (1985, 1991). In addition, analysis and evaluation of conceptual frameworks tend to be a frequent assignment for students in graduate nursing courses.

Although the approach to analysis and evaluation differs by author, the strengths and limitations of various conceptual frameworks are well documented in the literature. Overall, analysis and evaluation greatly increased awareness of conceptual frameworks as theoretical structures for nursing. However, analysis and evaluation also documented that data to support the validity of any conceptual framework were sparse (Fawcett, 1989; Fitzpatrick & Whall, 1989b; Moody, Wilson, Smyth, Tittle, & Vancott, 1988; Silva, 1986, 1987).

Validity addresses fundamental questions about the characteristics of knowledge, primarily what constitutes truth. The criteria most frequently used by philosophers to examine truth are correspondence, cohesion, and pragmatism (Silva & Sorrell, 1992). Validation is the process of examining "truth" or "goodness" on the basis of evidence. Validation is necessary to ensure that conceptual frameworks are not accepted at face value or rejected out of hand (Fawcett, 1989).

Validation of nursing's conceptual and theoretical structures has been slow. One reason for this was undoubtedly the dominance of a positivist perspective of science. From a positivist perspective, validation was empirical only and judged by correspondence criteria of truth. Verification occurred by attempts at falsification via rigorous testing. Both the publications by Silva (1986) and Acton, Irvin, and Hopkins (1991) set forth evaluation criteria for theory testing research that reinforced this deductive and quantitative approach (Silva & Sorrell, 1992; Whall, 1989).

Although empirical testing is one approach to validation, there are others. The doorway to expanded perspectives of validating conceptual frameworks was opened by Fawcett (1984) and Fitzpatrick and Whall (1983) in the early 1980s. Fawcett clearly stressed the need to determine the credibility of conceptual models.[2] Because conceptual models are too broad and abstract to be directly tested, they must be linked with other theories. Fawcett called these created structures "conceptual-theoretical systems." Others refer to these less abstract, more specific theories as "middle range."

In terms of credibility, the initial step was to examine the logical congruence of the borrowed theories with the nursing conceptual model (Whall, 1980). Borrowed theories could be from nursing or

other disciplines. Additional steps in examining credibility depend
on whether the conceptual-theoretical system is to be used in research, education, administration, or clinical practice (Fawcett, 1989).
For example, research findings constitute an indirect test of the
credibility of the conceptual model. Fawcett's criteria for evaluating
research were adapted from Silva (1986).

In clinical practice, credibility of the conceptual-theoretical system can be indirectly examined on the basis of the outcome of nursing care. Several steps were identified. First, prototypical conceptual-
theoretical systems are developed for specific patient groups. Care is
individualized and provided on the basis of nursing process guidelines suggested by each conceptual model. Credibility is examined in
terms of expected patient outcomes. Outcomes would be specific to
and congruent with the focus or goal of the model.

Other considerations that informally contribute to determination
of the credibility of conceptual models are social significance and
appropriateness of the fit between the nursing situation and the
model (Fawcett, 1989). Although the criteria for examining social
significance and fit are not as specific as the steps for evaluating
research, Fawcett identified that they could be used to evaluate
published reports of nursing practice. In 1992, further support for,
and clarification of the use of, conceptual models in practice, particularly the importance of data in evaluating credibility of conceptual
models, was published (Fawcett, 1992).

Whall (1989), in the second edition of *Conceptual Models of
Nursing: Analysis and Application* (Fitzpatrick & Whall, 1989a), also
addressed the validity of conceptual frameworks in her discussion of
"empirical examination." Drawing from the work of Ellis (1984),
Suppe and Jacox (1985), Benner (1984), Carper (1978), and Meleis
(1985), Whall suggested several ways to examine nursing conceptual
models,[3] which she described as products of the discipline. These included (a) research conceptualized within a conceptual model, (b) research on concepts and relationships found within a conceptual
model, (c) research examination of statements derived from conceptual models, and (d) examination of conceptual models in practice.

Whall (1989) stated that two of these areas, research framed on or
related to a conceptual model and practice applications, had not consistently been considered useful for the discipline. Although research

framed with a conceptual model does not directly or indirectly test the conceptual model, it does, however, place phenomena within the context of nursing. Taken together and over time, this could delineate distinct characteristics of nursing knowledge. According to Whall, practice applications that include examination of nursing process, health outcomes, and practice goals from conceptual models also contribute to the empirical value of a conceptual model, especially when examined for issues of adequacy and logical consistency.

When moving from conceptual models to more specific research and/or practice applications, faithfulness and congruency are important evaluation issues. Whall (1989) indicated that some flexibility is necessary to move the science of nursing forward:

> Nursing, as an art, has to do with skill gained either in research or practice. Remaining faithful to the model—to its concepts, relationships, and assumptions—is both a scientific process as well as an art. An important issue regarding nursing as an art concerns the view that one's artistic impression or application is free to vary from that of others, including a model's author or originator. Although one should be as clear as possible as to interpretations made or artistic license taken, these interpretations should be valued on their own merits and not solely on their congruence or faithfulness to a given model. In this way, each model could become a stimulus to further growth within the discipline, and not a restrictive influence. If nursing is to grow and develop as a science, original creations such as nursing conceptual models should be open to varied interpretations and free to develop in unrestricted fashion. (p. 8)

More recently, Silva and Sorrell (1992) expanded on testing nursing theory by identifying three additional approaches: critical reasoning, personal experiences, and application to practice. The discussion clearly supported the need to go beyond deductive testing and empirical evidence as the only approaches to knowing. Strengths of the ideas set forth by Silva and Sorrell were a clear focus on process and recognition of multiple philosophical views.

Despite some differences in terms and approaches, there is clear evidence of progress in recognizing the contributions that conceptual frameworks have made, and can make, in the development of nursing knowledge. Other events support and facilitate this important work.

One is publication of *Nursing Science Quarterly* in 1987, a journal dedicated to publishing original manuscripts focused on development, research, and practice related to existing nursing frameworks. Another significant factor is the appearance of "second-generation theorists," a description I use for persons who work from specific conceptual frameworks or theories. Notable examples are Susan Taylor, who works from Orem's (1991) self-care theory, and Elizabeth Barrett and Violet Malinski, who work from Rogers's science of unitary human beings (Rogers, 1970). Second-generation theorists differ from original theorists, experts, and scholars in analysis and evaluation and from the many nurses who use conceptual frameworks to guide practice. Like original theorists and analysis and evaluation experts, second-generation theorists have a firm foundation in philosophy of science, nursing science, and theory from other disciplines. Unlike the intent of nurses who use conceptual framework in practice, the intent of second-generation theorists is far beyond application to extension, evaluation, clarification, and overall advancement of conceptual-theoretical structures and, consequently, of nursing knowledge.

In this text, we use the phrase "advancing nursing science" to encompass what others have referred to as extending, examining, evaluating, and validating knowledge developed from nursing's conceptual frameworks and theories. This includes empirical testing as well as more quantitative approaches. The need for a broader perspective is supported in the nursing literature as both appropriate and necessary given the abstract nature of nursing's conceptual-theoretical structures.

The focus of this text is advancing nursing knowledge based on Imogene King's systems framework for nursing. Imogene King is recognized as one of the pioneers in conceptual-theoretical nursing. Her early interest in the area was linked to development of conceptual frameworks for nursing curriculum.

> Writings in the mid-1960s (King, 1964) expressed ideas about the need for focus, organization, and use of nursing's knowledge base. In 1968, King wrote of a conceptual frame of reference for nursing based on the concepts of perception, communication, interpersonal relationships, health, and social institutions. A conceptual

framework for nursing (organized around personal, interpersonal, social systems, and the concepts of perception, information, energy, interpersonal relationships, communication, social organization, role, and status) was published in *Toward a Theory for Nursing* (1971). The goal in developing the framework was to address the essence of nursing and move toward a general systems theory for nursing (King, 1971).

Refinements and changes in King's conceptual framework were made during the 1970s. In 1981, *A Theory for Nursing: Systems, Concepts, Process* was published. That text reflected reformulation of person and environment, refinement of the open system's orientation, expanded concepts for understanding systems and their interactions and, overall, a more formalized conceptual framework. In addition, King presented the theory of goal attainment derived from the conceptual framework. That 1981 text served as the primary source for learning about, studying, and critiquing King's work for over a decade.

Over the years, King has provided explanation, clarification, and expansion of concepts for what is now referred to as a systems framework for nursing. King has addressed questions and concerns raised by others (Fawcett, 1989; Gonot, 1989; Magan, 1987; Meleis, 1991) and has affirmed a strong belief in the enduring nature of her perspective over time and for the 21st century (King, personal communication, February 20, 1994). (Frey, in press)[4]

In addition to publications by King, there have been publications about her framework and theory of goal attainment written by others. Several analysis and evaluation critiques have been published (Ackermann et al., 1994; Fawcett, 1989; Frey, in press; Meleis, 1991). King's work was not included in Silva's (1986) review of research testing nursing theory because it did not meet inclusion criteria of at least six published empirical studies (Silva, 1987). Although Silva included only empirical studies, the number of nonempirical publications citing King's framework at that time was small. In the past 5 to 6 years there has been an increase in the number of publications based on King's framework and theory, especially in the areas of theory development, testing, and use in practice. In addition to work done in the United States, there has been considerable interest in King's work in other countries. This includes several excellent hospital-based practice applications in Canada, a replication study in Japan, and concept development in Sweden (Frey, in press). Two theories have been derived from the systems framework and published in the literature. The better known is King's own theory of goal attainment, published in 1981 as noted. The second is Frey's (1989) formulation of families, children, and chronic illness.

In 1989, I first discussed with King my work with extending the systems framework to a middle-range theory. Over the next few years, King provided the names of persons who worked with her framework and theory, many of whom had been her students or who otherwise had contacted her directly. Additional contacts with others interested in King's work were made through professional organizations and meetings, schools of nursing with graduate programs, and literature searches. Over a period of several years, it became increasingly clear that there were a number of nurses actively working with both King's framework and her theory. The work being done by the group was quite diverse in terms of approach, clinical populations, and substantive focus. With limited exceptions, few had published their work. The interest in and commitment to advancing nursing knowledge from King's systems framework for nursing has served as the driving force to publish this text.

In the remaining chapters in Part I, Dr. King presents her perspective of nursing and science, as well as a summary of her systems framework and theory of goal attainment. It is assumed that readers will have read, or concomitantly read, King's 1981 text. King's pre- and post-1981 writings are strongly recommended for a more comprehensive understanding of her work.

Chapters in Parts II and III address advancement of the systems framework and theory of goal attainment, respectively. Organization of Parts II and III was based on the authors' starting point (systems framework or theory) rather than on their approach to knowledge development. This was a deliberate decision by the editors after identifying that considerable work had been done with each. Finally, in Part IV, Jacqueline Fawcett and Ann Whall, both recognized leaders in nursing models and theories, provide an evaluation of the progress of knowledge development to date as well as direction for the future.

It is hoped that this text will not only reflect the contribution to nursing science from King's systems framework and theory of goal attainment but also serve as a model for others who choose to advance nursing science from a nursing conceptual framework. This approach to knowledge development should further define nursing's unique contribution to health and health care in the 21st century.

Notes

1. I prefer to use the term *framework* rather than *model*.
2. Fawcett prefers to use the term *model* rather than *framework*.
3. Whall prefers to use the term *model* rather than *framework*.
4. An expanded version of this material appears in Frey (in press). The section quoted here is reprinted by permission from Appleton & Lange.

References

Ackermann, M. L., Brink, S. A., Clanton, J. A., Jones, C. G., Marriner-Tomey, A., Moody, S. L., Perlich, G. L., Price, D. L., & Prusinski, B. B. (1994). Theory of goal attainment. In A. Marriner-Tomey (Ed.), *Nursing theorists and their work* (pp. 305-322). St. Louis, MO: C. V. Mosby.

Acton, G. J., Irvin, B. L., & Hopkins, B. A. (1991). Theory-testing research: Building the science. *Advances in Nursing Science, 14*(1), 52-61.

Benner, P. (1984). *From novice to expert: Excellence and power in clinical nursing practice.* Menlo Park, CA: Addison-Wesley.

Carper, B. A. (1978). Fundamental patterns of knowing in nursing. *Advances in Nursing Science, 1*(1), 13-23.

Ellis, R. (1984, October). *Theory development in nursing: The state of the art.* Paper presented at the 50th Anniversary Celebration of the Sir Mortimer Davis Jewish General Hospital, Montreal, Quebec.

Fawcett, J. (1983). Hallmarks of success in nursing theory development. In P. L. Chinn (Ed.), *Advances in nursing theory development* (pp. 3-17). Rockville, MD: Aspen.

Fawcett, J. (1984). *Analysis and evaluation of conceptual models of nursing.* Philadelphia: F. A. Davis.

Fawcett, J. (1989). *Analysis and evaluation of conceptual models of nursing* (2nd ed.). Philadelphia: F. A. Davis.

Fawcett, J. (1992). Conceptual models and nursing practice: The reciprocal relationship. *Journal of Advanced Nursing, 17,* 224-228.

Fitzpatrick, J. J., & Whall, A. L. (1983). *Conceptual models of nursing: Analysis and application.* Norwalk, CT: Appleton & Lange.

Fitzpatrick, J. J., & Whall, A. L. (1989a). *Conceptual models of nursing: Analysis and application* (2nd ed.). Norwalk, CT: Appleton & Lange.

Fitzpatrick, J. J., & Whall, A. L. (1989b). Guidelines for analysis of nursing's conceptual models. In J. Fitzpatrick & A. Whall (Eds.), *Conceptual models of nursing: Analysis and application* (2nd ed., pp. 23-31). Norwalk, CT: Appleton & Lange.

Frey, M. A. (1989). Social support and health: A theoretical formulation derived from King's conceptual framework. *Nursing Science Quarterly, 2,* 138-148.

Frey, M. A. (in press). Imogene M. King's conceptual framework of nursing. In J. J. Fitzpatrick & A. L. Whall (Eds.), *Conceptual models of nursing: Analysis and application* (3rd ed.). Norwalk, CT: Appleton & Lange.

Frey, M. A., Rooke, L., Sieloff, C., Messmer, P. R., & Kameoka, T. (in press). Advancement of King's framework in Japan, Sweden, and the United States. *Image: Journal of Nursing Scholarship.*

Gonot, P. J. (1989). Imogene M. King's conceptual framework of nursing. In J. J. Fitzpatrick & A. L. Whall (Eds.), *Conceptual models of nursing: Analysis and application* (2nd ed., pp. 271-283). Norwalk, CT: Appleton & Lange.

Hempel, C. G. (1952). *Fundamentals of concept formation in empirical science.* Chicago: University of Chicago Press.

Huch, M. H. (1988). Theory based practice: Structuring nursing care. *Nursing Science Quarterly, 1*(1), 6-7.

King, I. M. (1964). Nursing theory: Problems and prospect. *Nursing Science, 2,* 394-403.

King, I. M. (1968). A conceptual framework of reference for nursing. *Nursing Research, 17*(1), 27-31.

King, I. M. (1971). *Toward a theory for nursing.* New York: John Wiley.

King, I. M. (1981). *A theory for nursing: Systems, concepts, process.* New York: John Wiley.

Magan, S. J. (1987). A critique of King's theory. In R. R. Parse (Ed.), *Nursing science: Major paradigms, theories, and critiques* (pp. 115-133). Philadelphia: W. B. Saunders.

Meleis, A. I. (1985). *Theoretical nursing: Development and progress.* New York: J. B. Lippincott.

Meleis, A. I. (1991). *Theoretical nursing: Development and progress* (2nd ed.). New York: J. B. Lippincott.

Moody, L. E., Wilson, M. E., Smyth, K., Tittle, M., & Vancott, M. L. (1988). Analysis of a decade of nursing practice research: 1977-1986. *Nursing Research, 37,* 374-379.

Nicoll, L. H. (1992). *Perspectives on nursing theory* (2nd ed.). Philadelphia: J. B. Lippincott.

Orem, D. E. (1991). *Nursing: Concepts of practice* (4th ed.). St. Louis, MO: Mosby Year Book.

Parse, R. R. (1987). *Nursing science: Major paradigms, theories, and critiques.* Philadelphia: W. B. Saunders.

Phillips, J. R. (1988). The reality of nursing research. *Nursing Science Quarterly, 1,* 48-49.

Reilly, D. E. (1975). Why a conceptual framework? *Nursing Outlook, 23,* 566-569.

Rogers, M. E. (1970). *An introduction to the theoretical basis of nursing.* Philadelphia: F. A. Davis.

Silva, M. C. (1986). Research testing nursing theory. *Advances in Nursing Science, 9*(1), 1-11.

Silva, M. C. (1987). Conceptual models of nursing. In J. J. Fitzpatrick & R. L. Taunton (Eds.), *Annual review of nursing research* (Vol. 5, pp. 229-246). New York: Springer.

Silva, M. C., & Sorrell, J. M. (1992). Testing of nursing theory: Critique and philosophical expansion. *Advances in Nursing Science, 14*(4), 12-23.

Smith, M. C. (1992). The distinctiveness of nursing knowledge. *Nursing Science Quarterly, 5,* 148-149.

Suppe, F., & Jacox, A. (1985). Philosophy of science and the development of nursing theory. In H. H. Werley & J. J. Fitzpatrick (Eds.), *Annual review of nursing research* (Vol. 3, pp. 241-263). New York: Springer.

Visintainer, M. A. (1986). The nature of knowledge and theory in nursing. *Image: Journal of Nursing Scholarship, 18*(2), 32-38.

Whall, A. L. (1980). Congruence between existing theories of family functioning and nursing theories. *Advances in Nursing Science, 3*(1), 59-67.

Whall, A. L. (1989). Nursing science: The process and products. In J. Fitzpatrick & A. Whall (Eds.), *Conceptual models of nursing: Analysis and application* (2nd ed., pp. 1-14). Norwalk, CT: Appleton & Lange.

$$\cdot\!\!\!\!-\!\!\!\!-\ 2\ -\!\!\!\!-\!\!\cdot$$

A Systems
Framework for Nursing

IMOGENE M. KING

$\mathbf{M}$**any ideas about the possibilities** of the 21st century have been published by futurists. Some are related to technological advances, resulting in changes in our environment and the way we communicate and interact in a global society (King, 1994). For example, both the speed of travel and instant communication have influenced events in our lives. We live in an information-based economy. Naisbitt (1982) notes that "we are bombarded with information but starved for knowledge" (p. 17). The world is experiencing an information technology revolution (Halal, 1992). Within these changes, one factor remains; that human beings interacting with their environments represent an ongoing process relative to life and health.

Author's Note: Portions of this chapter were previously published in *Toward a Theory for Nursing: General Concepts of Human Behavior* (New York: John Wiley, 1971) and in *A Theory for Nursing: Systems, Concepts, Process* (Albany, NY: Delmar Publishers, 1981) and are reproduced by permission.

Transitory changes have permeated our lives. Although change is a continuous process, a few characteristics have remained an integral part of nursing practice. Nursing continues to be a helping profession providing a service that meets a social need. A part of this service is to give care to individuals and groups who are acutely and moderately ill. Nurses are the constant persons in the health care delivery system. They give care to individuals who have chronic diseases and need rehabilitation to help them use their potential ability to function as human beings. Nurses offer guidance and counseling for individuals and groups to help them maintain health. Nurses are partners with physicians, allied health professionals, and families in promoting health, preventing disease, and managing care for individuals and groups.

A part of the service provided by nurses deals with specific skills that they are expected to possess. Two such skills, observation and communication, are important for collecting reliable and valid information to make decisions by which to implement a plan of care. Some of nursing functions have not changed. However, some nursing tasks have been delegated to nonprofessional personnel, and nurses have assumed more physician-delegated and hospital management activities. Because my systems framework has been synthesized from basic elements in nursing, it will persist into the 21st century despite professional and social changes. This framework provides structure; introduces learners to basic theoretical knowledge and ways of thinking, both inductively and deductively; and helps individuals value their own thinking and feelings.

Functions of a Conceptual Framework

In *general*, functions of a framework include the following:

- To provide a way to organize a multitude of facts into meaningful wholes
- To provide a common theoretical basis for communication about perceived relationships in a field of study
- To direct attention to processes and relationships

- To guide one to look for, and consider, specific facts
- To provide a way to order knowledge for use in a variety of situations

For nursing *specifically*, the functions of a conceptual framework include:

- To provide a basic organizing focus for the domain of nursing
- To provide a system for classifying the knowledge, skills, and values of nursing as a discipline
- To provide a way of ordering facts into a system that organizes nursing's subject matter into a whole system
- To show relationships in the concepts and processes essential for teaching and for practicing nursing

A Systems Framework for Nursing Theory

Language and semantics influence the communication and perception of individuals and groups. Words are the vehicles we use to express our ideas. When we explain our ideas, we are sharing our concepts with persons in our environment. A concept is a representation of each person's knowledge of his or her world—that is, his or her reality.

Concepts give meaning to our sense perceptions and permit generalizations about persons, objects, and things. They are abstractions from our concrete experiences stored in our memories and recalled for use at later points in time. Concepts are the building blocks of cognition and represent one's substantive knowledge. They offer one approach to describe a common language that provides knowledge of multiple facts in a profession (King, 1988).

> Nurses use words, gestures, and actions to communicate information and to establish relationships with many individuals in nursing situations. Analysis of word symbols and of natural situations provides a way to identify underlying concepts that have meaning for nurses and for the recipient of care and that assist in identifying basic elements in nursing practice. (King, 1971, p. 21)

My analysis of the nursing literature, which spans more than a 20-year period, provided a list of terms used by nurses to describe nursing. This initial list of words was organized into more comprehensive concepts. Subsequently, I reviewed many years of research in, and outside of, nursing relative to the concepts. My observations of practicing nurses showed me that knowledge of these concepts was being used to plan and give care to individuals and families.

In the late 1960s, study of systems research gave me knowledge of general systems theory and operations research. This information helped me visualize nursing as the most complex profession in the health care field and raised several questions: What is the goal of nursing? What are the functions of nurses? How can nurses continue to expand their knowledge to provide quality care?

Developing one's concepts is one approach to ensure continuous learning in one's lifetime. My framework answers many other questions related to nursing's goals and functions.

In my initial thoughts about theory and nursing, I identified three major problems: (a) the lack of a professional language, (b) an antitheoretical bias, and (c) that the domain of nursing had not yet been identified (King, 1964). These problems, cited 30 years ago, have been partially resolved in the 1990s.

A frame of reference for the domain of nursing was published (King, 1968). Some of my original ideas in 1968 were expanded into a systems framework for nursing (King, 1971) in a book that received the 1973 Book of the Year Award from the *American Journal of Nursing.*

My systems framework was formulated to serve several purposes. First, it provides a way of thinking about the "real world" of nursing practice. Second, it suggests one approach for selecting concepts from the literature that represent fundamental knowledge for the practice of professional nursing. Third, it shows a process for developing concepts that symbolize experiences within various environments in which nursing is practiced. Although a conceptual framework is abstract, the concepts represent knowledge that can be used in concrete situations.

A framework serves as a means of communication. In any discussion of the nature of nursing, the focus revolves around human beings interacting with their environment. Human behavior is composed of human acts, process, and actions. "Nursing acts, like all human acts, are a sequence of behaviors of interacting persons who recognize a situation, and the activities related to it, and usually exert some control over the events to achieve goals" (King, 1971, p. 24). This process is a series of acts that connote action. "A nursing situation is conceived to be the immediate environment, spatial and temporal reality, in which nurses and the recipients of care establish relationships to cope with health states and adjust to changes in activities of daily living if the situation demands it" (King, 1971, p. 24).

The framework shown in Figure 2.1 demonstrates one approach to studying systems as a whole rather than as isolated parts of a system. In performing their functions, nurses interact with individuals and groups in a variety of health care systems. The framework shows three levels of interactions in any social system in which human beings are the focus (King, 1981).

The unit of analysis in this framework is human behavior in a variety of social environments. Each individual is a personal system. Individuals interact in groups that represent interpersonal systems that may consist of two or three persons or that may be classified as small and large groups. Groups are formed as social systems in a community within a society. This framework describes environments within which human beings grow, develop, and perform daily activities. The concepts in the framework are the organizing dimensions and represent knowledge essential for understanding the interactions between the three systems. The concepts of self, body image, growth and development, perception, learning, time, and personal space were placed in the personal systems because this knowledge relates to individuals. The concepts that emphasize interactions between two or more persons were placed in the interpersonal systems. Verbal and nonverbal communication, interaction, stress, role, and transaction provide essential knowledge for nurses in working with individuals, families, and small and large groups. Concepts that provide knowledge for nurses to function in larger systems were placed in social systems. Concepts of decision making, organization, power, authority, and status represent essential knowledge for nurses to function in their professional role.

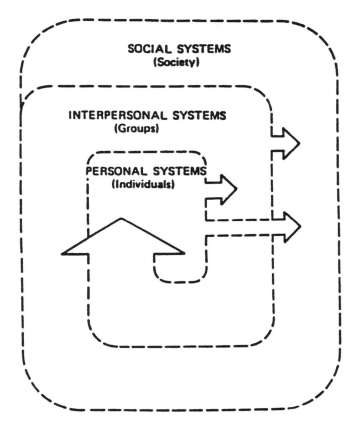

Figure 2.1. King's Conceptual Framework for Nursing
SOURCE: From *A Theory for Nursing: Systems, Concepts, Process*, p. 11, by I. M. King, 1981. Copyright © 1981 by Delmar Publishers. Reprinted by permission of the publisher.

The concepts in the framework are not limited to only one of the dynamic interacting systems but cut across all three systems. Knowledge of all of the concepts is used in most nursing situations.

Analysis of the nursing literature has shown that many nurses have used knowledge of these concepts. Nurses indicate that this framework gives them a greater awareness of the knowledge they use in their practice. In addition, they now have words to describe and explain nursing to others (Carter & Dufour, 1994). Nurses have discussed ways they have used knowledge of personal space to understand a patient's behavior in hospitals. Knowledge of perception has helped them understand patient and family perceptions and prevented potential conflict in some situations. Nurses have become aware that their nonverbal behavior speaks louder than their words.

The systems framework discussed here was defined in nursing as the dynamic interactions and essential components used by nurses to identify and achieve goals. For example, "The dynamics of nursing can be described as a constant restructuring of relationships between nurse and client to cope with existential problems and to learn ways of adjusting to changes in daily activities" (King, 1971, p. 103). "It is the nurse in a health care system who relates knowledge, skills, technology, values and administrative structure into a unified approach for delivering nursing and health care within social systems" (King, 1971, pp. 63, 103).

"The goal of nursing is to help individuals and groups attain, maintain, and restore health. In nursing situations where the goal of life and health cannot be achieved, as in a terminal illness, nurses give care and help individuals die with dignity" (King, 1971, p. 84). Nurses play strategic roles in the process of human growth and development and in helping individuals cope with episodes of illness in the life cycle. They have an essential role in community planning for the delivery of health services to the public. "As professionals, nurses deal with behavior of individuals and groups in potentially stressful situations related to health and illness and help them learn how to cope with daily living" (King, 1971, p. 84).

My framework has been used by faculty groups as the organizing dimension for building and/or reorganizing curricula in an undergraduate program (Daubenmire, 1989, p. 167), and faculty members in associate and master's degree programs have also used this framework (King, 1986). Several nurse administrators have indicated their use of this systems approach to identify goals, functions, and resource allocations to make decisions in the nursing department (King, 1989).

Summary

My systems framework has described a holistic view of the complexity in nursing, within various groups, in different types of health care systems. The concepts provide knowledge that helps one analyze the relations between individuals as personal systems and between small and large groups as interpersonal systems, interacting in a variety of social groups called social systems. This framework differs from other conceptual schema in that it is concerned not with fragmenting human beings and the environment but with human transactions in different types of environments. This framework exhibits the characteristics of open systems: goals, structure, functions, resources, and decision making. Several theories have been derived from the framework. One, the theory of goal attainment, is presented in the next chapter.

References

Carter, K. F., & Defour, L. T. (1994). King's theory: A critique of the critiques. *Nursing Science Quarterly, 7*(3), 128-133.

Daubenmire, M. J. (1989). A baccalaureate nursing curriculum based on King's conceptual framework. In J. Riehl-Sisca (Ed.), *Conceptual models for nursing practice* (3rd ed., pp. 167-178). Norwalk, CT: Appleton & Lange.

Halal, W. E. (1992). The information technology revolution. *The Futurist, 26*(4), 10-15.

King, I. M. (1964). Nursing theory: Problems and prospects. *Nursing Science, 2*(5), 395-403.

King, I. M. (1968). A conceptual frame of reference. *Nursing Research, 17*(1), 27-31.

King, I. M. (1971). *Toward a theory for nursing.* New York: John Wiley.

King, I. M. (1981). *A theory for nursing: Systems, concepts, process.* New York: Delmar.

King, I. M. (1986). *Curriculum and instruction in nursing.* Norwalk, CT: Appleton-Century-Crofts.

King, I. M. (1988). Concepts: Essential elements in theories. *Nursing Science Quarterly, 1*(1), 22-25.

King, I. M. (1989). King's systems framework for nursing administration. In B. Henry, C. Arndt, M. Di Vincenti, & A. Marriner-Tomey (Eds.), *Dimensions of nursing administration: Theory, research, education, practice* (pp. 35-53). Boston: Blackwell.

King, I. M. (1994). Quality of life and goal attainment. *Nursing Science Quarterly, 7*(1), 29-32.

Naisbitt, J. (1982). *Megatrends.* New York: Warner.

The Theory of Goal Attainment

IMOGENE M. KING

In the past, science reduced phenomena to small elementary units for the purpose of studying parts of phenomena. In the last half of the 20th century, a revolution has occurred in philosophy of science. For example, scientists, concerned with the "wholeness" of phenomena, developed new ideas and approaches for studying human behavior. General systems theory was created for sciences concerned with "organized wholes." Von Bertalanffy (1968) noted that "general system theory is a general science of wholeness" (p. 37). This scientific movement gave me hope that one could study the complexity of nursing as an "organized whole." My systems framework was designed to explain organized wholes within which nurses are expected to function. The multiple variables that influence perceptions, roles, responsibilities, and decision making in a variety of health care systems and in working with families require a conceptualization of

Author's Note: Portions of this chapter were previously published in *Toward a Theory for Nursing: General Concepts of Human Behavior* (New York: John Wiley, 1971) and in *A Theory for Nursing: Systems, Concepts, Process* (Albany, NY: Delmar Publishers, 1981) and are reproduced by permission.

the whole. However, one cannot study the universe as a whole. One must develop theories to study whole systems within the universe. My framework of dynamic interacting systems provided a comprehensive structure from which I developed a theory for nursing.

Several guidelines about the functions of theory can be identified from the literature. Theory is a way of discovering new knowledge in any field of study and offers ways of thinking about phenomena. It is a way of looking at facts, organizing them into a system, and finding new relationships. Theory provides reference points from which to describe, explain, and predict events in our world. It guides us to collect facts in a systematic way, to formulate hypotheses to test, to ask questions to be answered, and to extend the range of knowledge useful in a profession. Theory is a way of systematizing and unifying knowledge, and it identifies gaps in knowledge in a discipline. Theories suggest ways to verify knowledge about decision making and provide a rationale for gathering reliable and valid data. Scientific knowledge for nursing is discovered through theory development and testing by means of research. Kaplan (1964) stated the "why" of theory: "Theories are not just means to other ends, and certainly not just to ends outside the scientific enterprise, but they may also serve as ends in themselves—to provide understanding which may be prized for its own sake" (p. 310).

A Theory for Nursing

The complexity and variety in health care systems demonstrate a need to organize knowledge for nursing by developing theories. The complexity in nursing is obvious when one attempts to define a human being interacting with other human beings in different types of environments.

The goal of my nursing system, as a whole, is health for individuals; health for groups, such as the family; and health for communities within a society. The means to attain goals at each level of the three dynamic interacting systems (personal, interpersonal, and social) are different. Nurses are the key persons in the health care system who identify the goals and the means to help individuals and families attain goals.

The theory of goal attainment exhibits the characteristics of a general systems theory: goal(s), structure, functions, resources, and decision making. The *goal* of the theory is represented in the concept of health, which includes health promotion, health maintenance, and regaining health when there is some interference along the life cycle—for example, an illness (King, 1990). In working to attain the goal of health, nurses provide care for the ill and disabled. They care for individuals who are dying. They provide support for families.

Structure is viewed as semipermeable boundaries between individuals, groups, and society. Structure provides a way of organizing large systems to work toward goal attainment for individuals and families. Structure indicates who is responsible for allocation of resources to enable persons to perform their functions. As we move into the 21st century, a systems approach is one way to cope with continuous technological changes to achieve system goals. The flow of information through communication, at all levels, is essential for goal attainment.

Functions in a system flow from goals and structure. Functions are carried out by individuals and groups within systems. Functions are usually specified and assigned to individuals, such as professional nurses.

Resources are essential to perform functions within a structure to attain goals. Technology and money are two types of resources needed in a health care system. Human beings are also a major resource in health care. When there is a decrease in human resources, one questions how goals can be attained.

Decision making is a vital characteristic in any health care setting —for example, in a hospital setting, who makes what decisions at each level of the framework I have developed. Decisions at one level of function influence the behavior of individuals at all levels and are reflected in outcomes—that is, in goals attained.

The Theory of Goal Attainment

The theory of goal attainment was derived from my open-systems framework. One question that motivated me to develop a theory was, What is the nature of nursing? When searching for the nature of something, one looks for its essence. The concepts in the personal and interpersonal systems and the role and decision-making concepts in social systems were selected because they are key components in the interactions of human beings with their environments. Nurses are first, and foremost, human beings who perform their functions in a professional role. It is the way in which nurses, in their role, do with and for individuals that differentiates nursing from other health professionals.

Nursing acts and actions provide a basic unit of analysis in the nursing process. In a nursing situation, a basic unit of behavior was identified as interactions between a nurse and a recipient of care. These phenomena are identified through knowledge of the major concepts of the theory, such as perception, communication, interaction, and transaction. Decision making is implicit for the interactions to take place. Testing the interrelationships of the concepts in nursing situations using qualitative and quantitative research methods has shown these concepts to be essential knowledge for nursing.

The criteria used to develop this theory are as follows:

1. What are the philosophical assumptions?
2. Are the concepts clearly identified and defined?
3. Are the concepts related in propositional statements or models?
4. Does the theory generate questions and hypotheses to be tested in research to generate knowledge and to affirm the theory?

These same criteria can be used to evaluate the theory.

Philosophical Assumptions. My assumptions about human beings are that they are open systems in transaction with the environment. Transaction connotes that there is no separateness between human beings and environment. Characteristics that are common to human beings are that they are unique, holistic individuals of intrinsic worth who are capable of rational thinking and decision making in most situations. Individuals are sentient and social, as observed by their interactions with persons and objects in the environment. They are perceived as reacting beings who are controlling, purposeful, action oriented, and time oriented in their behavior (King, 1981). "Individuals have the capacity to think, to know, to make choices, and to select alternative courses of actions. Human beings have the ability through their language and other symbols to record their history and to preserve their culture" (King, 1986, p. 56).

Individuals differ in their needs, wants, and goals. Because each person is unique, the nature of values emanates from the nature of human beings. Values form the basis for each person's goals. They are demonstrated in the standards of human conduct and have been handed down from one generation to another. Values are linked to cultures and, therefore, vary from person to person, family to family, and society to society. When there is disagreement between two or more individuals, value conflict may occur. When one is pressured to make choices, intrapersonal conflict in values may occur.

> Nurses play strategic roles in the process of human growth and development and in helping individuals cope with disturbances in their health. . . . As professionals, nurses deal with behavior of individuals and groups in potentially stressful situations, pertaining to health, illness, and crises, and help people cope with changes in daily activities. (King, 1981, p. 13)

Nursing is perceiving, thinking, relating, judging, and acting vis-à-vis the behavior of individuals who come to a health care system. A nursing situation is the immediate environment, spatial and temporal reality, in which two individuals establish a relationship to cope with events in the situation.

Concepts. The concepts of the theory selected from my framework are self, perception, communication, interaction, transaction, growth and development, stress, time, personal space, and role. These concepts provided substantive knowledge for nursing. A few of the concepts were used to design a model of transactions in which decisions are implicit. The human process of interactions formed the basis for designing a model (see Figure 3.1) of transactions that depicts theoretical knowledge used by nurses to help individuals and groups attain goals (King, 1981, p. 61).

This process model identifies the nature of nurse-client interactions that lead to goal attainment. Two people (nurse and a client) who are usually strangers meet in a health care environment to help

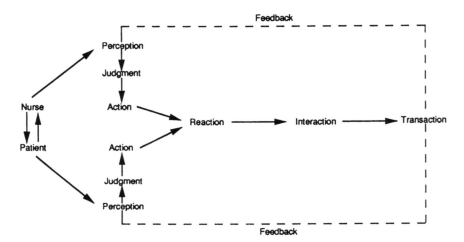

Figure 3.1. A Model of Nurse-Patient Transactions
SOURCE: From *A Theory for Nursing: Systems, Concepts, Process*, p. 61, by I. M. King, 1981. Copyright © 1981 by Delmar Publishers. Reprinted by permission of the publisher.

and be helped, to maintain health that permits functioning in roles. This process demonstrates that nurses interact with clients purposefully to mutually set goals and explore and agree on the means to attain the goals. Mutual goal setting is based on (a) nurses' assessment of a client's concerns, problems, and disturbances in health; (b) nurses' and client's perceptions of the interference; and (c) their sharing information whereby each functions to help the client attain the goals identified. In addition, nurses interact with family members when clients cannot verbally participate in goal setting. This process identifies behaviors in nurse-client interactions that lead to outcomes—that is, to goal attainment.

The process model of transactions is related to the nursing process called *method* (assess, plan, implement, and evaluate) in that the concepts provide theoretical knowledge to implement the method. The relationship between the nursing process as method and the nursing process as theory is shown in Table 3.1.

A concept of transaction is the valuational component of the human process of interactions. A concept of communication is the informational component of the human process of interactions.

TABLE 3.1   The Relationship Between Nursing Method and Nursing Theory

Nursing Process as Method	*Nursing Process as Theory*
A system of interrelated actions	A system of interrelated concepts
Assess	Perceptions of nurse and client
	Communication of nurse and client
	Interaction of nurse and client
Plan	Decision making about goals
	Explore means to attain goals
	Agree to means to attain goals
Implement	Transactions made
Evaluate	Goal attained (if not, why not)

SOURCE: From "King's Theory of Goal Attainment," by I. M. King, 1992, *Nursing Science Quarterly, 5*, 19-26. Copyright © 1992 by Chestnut House Publications. Reprinted with permission.

Propositions.   According to Dubin (1978), a proposition is a truth statement about a theory. Two examples in relation to the theory of goal attainment are the following:

> If perceptual congruence is present in nurse-client interactions, transactions will occur.
> If nurse and client make transactions in a nursing situation, goals will be attained. (King, 1981, p. 149)

In a critique of my framework and theory, Austin and Champion (1983) diagrammed positive and negative relationships between concepts. One of their examples is shown in Figure 3.2.

As shown in the diagram, perceptual accuracy (PA), role congruence (RCN), and communication (CM) between nurse and client lead to transactions (T). Transactions lead to growth and development (GD) and to goal attainment (GA). Goal attainment leads to satisfaction (S) and to effective nursing care (NCe) (Austin & Champion, 1983).

Hypotheses and Research Questions.   Because the term *transaction* was not a concept in the nursing literature at the time this theory

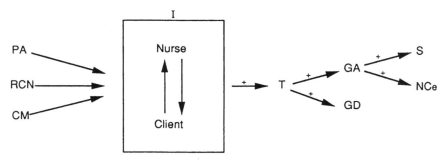

Figure 3.2. Relationships Between Concepts of the Theory
SOURCE: From "King's Theory for Nursing: Explication and Evaluation," p. 54, by J. K. Austin and V. L. Champion, 1983, in P. L. Chin (Ed.), *Advances in Nursing Theory Development*. Copyright © 1983 by Aspen System Corporation. Reprinted by permission of the publisher.

was developed, I conducted a study to answer the question, Are transactions observable in nurse-client interactions? Reliable and valid nurse-patient interaction data collected by another investigator were used to formulate an operational definition of transaction. The definition was used to identify transactions in my study. My small sample consisted of 17 cases of nurse-client interactions. Observers were trained and data collected using nonparticipant observations (King, 1981, pp. 150-156). The question was answered in the affirmative. That is, the nurses made a transaction in 12 of the cases. A classification system shown in Table 3.2 was constructed and may be used by nurses to evaluate their own care. Published and unpublished studies (e.g., those included in this volume) have been conducted to test other hypotheses and answer research questions about this theory.

The theory of goal attainment has been called a general systems theory because it is a set of elements joined together by communication links with goal-directed, purposeful behavior. When outcomes are stated in terms of goals to be attained by the recipient of care, nurses have a way to evaluate the effectiveness of their care. Goals set that lead to goals attained equals effective nursing care.

A goal-oriented record was developed to document goals set and goals attained. The major elements in this record system are (a) database, (b) nursing diagnosis, (c) goal list, (d) nursing orders, (e) flow

TABLE 3.2   A Classification System of Nurse-Patient Interactions That Lead to Transactions

- Action
- Reaction
- Disturbance
- Mutual goal setting
- Explore means to achieve goal
- Agree on means to achieve goal
- Transactions

SOURCE: From *A Theory for Nursing: Systems, Concepts, Process*, p. 156, by I. M. King, 1981. Copyright © 1981 by Delmar Publishers. Reprinted by permission of the publisher.

sheets, (f) progress notes, and (g) discharge summary. A reliable and valid assessment instrument provides information for the database. The assessment form includes a nursing history, activities of daily living, roles of client, stressors in the environment, patient perception, patient goals and values, and learning needs.

An opportunity was made available for me to engage in a continuing education program sponsored by the University of Maryland to develop an instrument to measure goal attainment. I learned very early on that my domain objectives had to be clearly specified. A goal attainment scale was developed and published (King, 1989, pp. 108, 117). This scale has been used by nurses as an assessment instrument in practice and in research.

Summary

Concepts from my systems framework were selected in developing the theory of goal attainment. Key concepts were then used to develop a model of transactions. Transactions lead to outcomes relative to energy expenditure, cost containment, and effective nursing care.

A goal-oriented nursing record system was designed to show the necessity for documenting nursing care that results in outcomes that are measurable. This record system facilitates the use of knowledge of the concepts in practice. This approach to documentation provides a way to measure outcomes that lead to quality improvement and cost containment in health care systems.

Knowledge of human behavior is essential to understand the nature of nursing whose focus is human-environment transactions. Thus knowledge of concepts helps nurses understand human behavior. The concept of transaction is the valuational component of the human process of interactions that lead to goal attainment and quality care. The many fine examples in this book demonstrate how some nurses have used the systems framework and theory in research, in education, in administration, and in practice.

References

Austin, J. K., & Champion, V. L. (1983). King's theory for nursing: Explication and evaluation. In P. L. Chin (Ed.), *Advances in nursing theory development* (pp. 49-62). Rockville, MD: Aspen.

Dubin, R. (1978). *Theory building.* New York: Free Press.

Kaplan, A. (1964). *A conduct of inquiry.* San Francisco, CA: Chandler.

King, I. M. (1981). *A theory for nursing: Systems, concepts, process.* New York: Delmar.

King, I. M. (1986). *Curriculum and instruction in nursing.* Norwalk, CT: Appleton-Century-Crofts.

King, I. M. (1989). Measuring health goal attainment in patients. In C. F. Waltz & O. L. Strickland (Eds.), *Measurement of nursing outcomes* (pp. 108-127). New York: Springer.

King, I. M. (1990). Health as the goal for nursing. *Nursing Science Quarterly,* 3(3), 123-128.

King, I. M. (1992). King's theory of goal attainment. *Nursing Science Quarterly,* 5(1), 19-26.

Von Bertalanffy, L. (1968). *General systems theory.* New York: George Braziller.

PART II

ADVANCING THE
SYSTEMS FRAMEWORK

·•—— **4** ——•·

A Systems View of Health

CYNTHIA KELSEY WINKER

The ancient Greeks viewed humanity as an integral part of nature. People and nature were seen as being subject to fixed organismic principles rather than to mystic and unpredictable influences (Smith, 1983). In the Greek culture, people were subject to teleological principles: "Hippocratic medical thought was based on the doctrine of the organic, teleological relation between the human body and the order of the universe of which it is a part" (Smith, 1983, p. 23). These rules or principles were believed by the Greeks to be appropriate to both people and nature. An understanding of these rules enabled one to understand health and also the relationship of illness to men and women.

As modern science began to develop, a mechanistic approach replaced the holistic and unitary science advocated by the Greeks. René Descartes (Cottingham, 1992) declared man to be *bête machine*, a mechanical beast. Sir Isaac Newton (1958) viewed the universe as an immense machine. French philosopher Julien Offray de La Mettrie (1748/1960) issued a declaration titled *L'Homme-machine* that contemplated humanity's machinelike instincts. William Harvey's (1847/1965) discovery that the heart functions as a pump was the advent of mechanical explanations for anatomical and physiological phenomena.

Although acknowledging that mechanistic, reductionistic thought had contributed significantly to advances in biomedical research, Ludwig Von Bertalanffy (1952, 1933/1962, 1967), father of general systems theory, denied the ability of these scientific paradigms to fully answer the questions posed by life and open systems. Von Bertalanffy further argued that even Descartes and Newton acknowledged the inadequacies of their science by declaring that these machines were created by God. However, much of medical science today remains reductionist in its approach, fostering the clinical model of health and creating the dichotomous approach to defining health as the absence of illness (Smith, 1983).

Although reductionism and mechanism are still popular models in the medical world, Smith (1983) believes a resurgence in Greek philosophy is present in health care today. In an important work published in 1983, Smith classifies four models of health: clinical, role performance, adaptive, and eudaimonistic. Smith defines eudaimonistic health as "the condition of complete development of the individual's potential. Illness is the condition that interrupts or obstructs this development" (p. 87). Eudaimonistic health considers the entire person. A full discussion of these four models is beyond the scope of this chapter; however, the eudaimonistic model will be relevant to this treatment of health within King's (1981) framework, for it is within that model that holism is associated with health.

The concept of holism is congruent with several principal schools of scientific thought. The one most relevant to this discussion is Ludwig Von Bertalanffy's (1933/1962) general systems theory. Von Bertalanffy rejected mechanism by saying, "Mechanism provides us with no grasp of the specific characteristics of organisms or the organization of organic processes among one another or the problem of the origin of organic 'teleology' " (Von Bertalanffy, 1933/1962, p. 46). Teleology is defined as the "explanation for phenomena by reference to some ultimate end for which a thing or event is produced" (Davidson, 1983, p. 78).

In addition to identifying the problem of teleology, Von Bertalanffy found no explanation in mechanistic thought to the phenomenon of equifinality. In general systems theory, the organism is considered to be active rather than reactive; therefore, equifinality is a critical characteristic that allows organisms to reach a final goal from different conditions in different ways (Von Bertalanffy, 1968a).

The biographer of Von Bertalanffy's life and work believed that in Von Bertalanffy's worldview, no room existed for humans to sit by as passive onlookers in "nature's game. But, because life is governed by the natural laws of systems, a successful participant must learn the rules" (Davidson, 1983, p. 95).

Von Bertalanffy (1981) said that we live as "denizen[s] of two worlds" (p. 17). One world is the biological world with traits or biological values that contribute to the survival of the species and of the individual. The other world is a world of human values that are behavioral or cultural and are associated with art, religion, and morals. The organism is manifest as form; the form functions in a culture; the culture and the individual decide on the meaningfulness of the symbols. For Von Bertalanffy, both biological and human value symbols must be intact for the survival of the individual and the species. Von Bertalanffy (1981) has said that human values are manifest in symbolic creations. Nurses are beginning to consider health and illness as human values (Huch, 1991).

King is a self-declared general systems theorist. Others who have reviewed her work have also categorized it as systems theory (Fawcett, 1989; Marriner-Tomey, 1989). Because King's (1981) theory is based in general systems theory, her definition of health can be critically analyzed using concepts from general systems theory. In particular, three concepts require review. A synthesis of these concepts into a new definition of health for use with King's theory will help nurses better care for a person as an open system. The three critical concepts are transformation, equifinality, and teleology.

Transformation

Most people have restricted their view of life because of the tendency to think of humans performing as machines in their biological responses to life. However, Von Bertalanffy believed that if the view one holds of life inspires awe, then one will treat life with reverence and each other with respect (Davidson, 1983). Bertalanffian science states that humans are open systems that interact with the environment; open systems are not just acted on. Nor do open systems simply react to an action. Crucial to Von Bertalanffy's view was the understanding that the organism is not a passive automaton reacting to stimuli but is for the most part an autonomously active system (Von Bertalanffy, 1952). Herein lies the problem.

Nursing science has, in the past, classified these biological responses as either adaptation or adjustment. We have not had a convenient label to apply to the real phenomenon. Prigogine and Stengers (1984) have supplied us with that missing term: *transformation*. Prigogine (Prigogine & Stengers, 1984) was able to further Von Bertalanffy's work in his theory of dissipative structures. He developed the idea that systems have upper and lower control limits in their ability to export entropy. The system will work within those limits until such time that a critical fluctuation occurs. When a critical fluctuation occurs, the boundaries of this fluctuation exceed the limits of the system. This brings the system to a bifurcation point. At the bifurcation point, the system will either fall into disorder or reorganize itself spontaneously. Because the process is out of control, the outcome is unpredictable. This transformation is seen by nurses when a person as an open system struggles between health and illness. This struggle is neither adaptation nor adjustment—concepts that are incongruent with general systems theory as originally conceived by Von Bertalanffy (1952, 1933/1962, 1967, 1968a, 1968b, 1981). Rather, the struggle is best understood as transformation, a concept consistent with general systems theory and directly related to the concepts of equifinality and teleology.

Equifinality

General systems theory views the phenomena of life as taking place in physical bodies that are "circumscribed in space" and thus seen in the "complex structure[s] that we call 'organisms' " (Von Bertalanffy, 1952, p. 11). These structures are "so ordered that they guarantee maintenance, construction, restitution, and reproduction" (p. 13). General systems theory does maintain that some biological phenomena are machinelike in their passive response to the environment. However, in large part, biological phenomenon are unmachinelike in that they are initiated from within the organism. This inner directedness is defined as *equifinality*. Equifinality is the "ability of the organism to reach a given final goal from different initial conditions and in different ways. [It is the] inner-directed ability of the organism to protect or restore its wholeness" (Davidson, 1983, p. 77). Von Bertalanffy's belief in equifinal self-preservation extends to the medical interventions that he believed frequently thwarted the body's natural healing powers (Davidson, 1983; Von Bertalanffy, 1976). Von Bertalanffy believed equifinality to be a basic characteristic of open systems and used that concept to link to the idea of teleology.

Teleology

Teleology has been debated as a metaphysical principle because it lacks testability. Teleology is the "explanation of phenomena by reference to some ultimate end for which a thing or event is believed to be produced" (Davidson, 1983, p. 227). Reading Von Bertalanffy's work first sparked in my mind the relationship of teleology to health and the absence of that relationship in King's concept of health. Later, after I read Judith Smith's (1983) work, the importance of teleology in conceptualizing health was confirmed.

As an open system, a person possesses the characteristic of teleology. Regarding the teleological nature of open systems, Von Bertalanffy (1933/1962) wrote:

> Whether we consider nutrition, voluntary and instinctive behaviors, development, the harmonious functioning of the organism under normal conditions, or its regulative functioning in cases of disturbances of the normal, we find that practically all vital processes are so organized that they are directed to the maintenance, production, or restoration of the wholeness of the organism. (p. 8)

Von Bertalanffy's ideas of teleology and wholeness are vital to King's nursing perspective, which considers the whole person as an open system.

King's Definition of Health

King (1981) has defined health as "dynamic life experiences of a human being, which implies continuous adjustment to stressors in the internal and external environment through optimum use of one's resources to achieve maximum potential for daily living. Illness is defined as a deviation from normal" (p. 5). King (1990) has also tied her view of health to role—that is, "Nurses help individuals and groups maintain their health so that they can function in their roles" (p. 127). She believes that the "goal [of nursing] is to help individuals maintain their health so they can function in their roles" (King, 1981, pp. 3-4).

I submit that role is but one of the symbols created out of our human values and, therefore, the restoration of role function or the main- tenance of role function, or both, is not the single goal of nursing. Von Bertalanffy (1981) believed that although the use of symbols separates humans from animals, symbols (e.g., money, status) are neither the reason for existence nor the sole purpose of the system. Von Bertalanffy (1933/1962) said that the "fundamental character of the living thing is organization" (p. 64). This being true, it follows that the system requires a complex organization of symbols created by both biological and human values.

In 1990, King revisited the concept of health. She found that in the general literature, health was seen as "relative, subjective, multidimensional, functional, and perceptual. . . . a state, a process, a diagnosis, a task, a response, or a goal" (pp. 124-125). In the nursing literature, King (1990) found health defined as a process, a functional state with both personal and subjective dimensions, and a continuum. In her original book in 1971, King stated that health "encompasses the whole man—physical, emotional, and social . . . within the cultural pattern in which he was born and to which he attempts to conform" (King, 1971, p. 67).

King does not believe that health is a linear process nor does she accept the dichotomy of health and illness on extremes of a continuum (King, 1971, 1981, 1990). However, she is not "encompass[ing] the whole man" when she limits health to being able to function in a role or "to achieve the maximum potential for daily living" (King, 1981, p. 5). Although she has written extensively on the subject of health over the past 25 years, it is interesting to note that she has not expanded her view.

King has been criticized for being mechanistic in her approach in the use of the terms *adaptation* and *adjustment* (Fawcett, 1989; Magan, 1987). She has also been criticized for limiting the definition of health to role function and the ability to participate in activities of daily living. Some have said caring for the dying patient is not compatible with King's definition of health (Meleis, 1991).

King's (1981) theory is meeting with success in nursing practice (Fawcett, 1989; Marriner-Tomey, 1989). However, to address the criticisms present today and to create understanding that is in congruence with general systems theory from which her work was derived, a new definition of health must be crafted. This definition development can be guided by the systems characteristics of teleology and equifinality in both the biological and human values symbolic world.

To expand King's definition of health, one can begin with the idea presented in her 1971 text: Health "encompasses the whole man— physical, emotional, and social . . . within the cultural pattern in which he was born and to which he attempts to conform" (King, 1971, p. 67). Taking this idea even further, one begins to understand that health is a value that is defined by the culture in which one lives and is expressed in symbols. One example of such a symbol is role and the ability to function in a role, but that is only one of many possible symbols.

As an open system, a person displays the characteristics of equifinality due to the teleological nature of the human system. Variations in the responses of the system are produced as a result of the interaction of the complex elements within the human system, which operates within the environment and the broader universe. These variations are manifest as diseases of the mind or body or alterations of various body systems. Dossey (1985) has suggested that health is evidence of our connection and interaction with the universe; and death is "a relentless shuttle between world of form and non form" (Dossey, 1985, p. 146). Therefore, limiting the definition of health to role function does not comprehend the interaction of people and the universe or the teleological nature of humanity.

The human system, because of its teleological nature, will strive to return to the aim for which the system was created. The role of the nurse is to understand the nature of this self-correcting system and plan interventions that allow the human system to move on to its desired end. From this point of view, individuals will have a different definition of health according to the symbols that have value for them or where the rules of nature are driving their system. The process is equifinal in nature in that, as Von Bertalanffy (1981) believed, human beings exhibit equifinal self-preservation. Too often, said Von Bertalanffy, the body's natural healing powers are interfered with by well-intentioned but harmful medical intervention (Davidson, 1983; Von Bertalanffy, 1976).

The nurse must realize and understand that persons as open systems are subject to "certain rules, rules that [are] appropriate to the nature of man. The knowledge of these rules is the most effective way to preserve health or recover from disease" (Smith, 1983, p. 25). The nurse can most effectively help patients by enabling them to identify those symbols in their lives that are of value to them. The nurse can then use equifinality and teleological principles to assist the restoration of the organism to wholeness with a minimum of interference. The goal of the nurse is to find meaningful symbols for patients depending on which way bifurcation has taken them. Because those outcomes are unpredictable, one cannot limit patients to being considered healthy if they can function in their roles; rather, health is present when the symbols that have meaning for patients are achieved. Those symbols could range from a return to role function or death with dignity.

Therefore, health is defined as the ability of the individual to create meaningful symbols based on either biological or human values within his or her cultural and individual value systems. The practice of nursing is aimed toward restoring or maximizing health through the mutual identification of symbols and the meaning attached to them, allowing the maximum expression in life or death.

This definition of health is consistent with two of the primary concepts in King's personal system: perception and self. King (1981) says that values "serve as organizing factors in one's perceptions" (p. 23). Perception is the foundation for creating an individual concept of self (King, 1981). Regarding self, King (1981) says:

> Knowledge of self is a key to understanding human behavior, because self is the way I define me to myself and to others. Self is all that I am. Self is what I think of me and what I am capable of being and doing. Self is subjective in that it is what I think I should be or would like to be. (p. 26)

King has also said that self is goal oriented. This inner directedness of self is congruent with the systems concepts of teleology and equifinality. King (1981) states that "the personal system is a unified, complex, whole self" (p. 27). In the personal system, perception and self can be thought of as products of an individual's human and biological values. Perception and self are expressed in the symbols humans create.

If we accept the prominence of health in the conceptual system, it follows that a definition of health consistent with general systems theory and true to the principles of King's (1981) systems framework must be crafted. The definition proposed in this chapter is consistent with the concepts and principles of general systems theory as conceived by Von Bertalanffy (1968a). This definition furthers King's work by broadening the definition, which allows it to be applied to all stages of growth and development of human beings.

King is to be commended for the work she has done. Her theory provides pragmatic direction for research and practice. The intent of offering this proposed definition of health is to enhance the logical congruence of her theory and to address criticisms that have been offered regarding the hint of mechanism in her work.

References

Cottingham, J. (1992). *The Cambridge companion to Descartes.* New York: Cambridge University Press.

Davidson, M. (1983). *Uncommon sense. The life and thought of Ludwig Von Bertalanffy*. Los Angeles: Tarcher.

Dossey, L. (1985). *Space, time, & medicine*. Boston: Shambala.

Fawcett, J. (1989). *Analysis and evaluation of conceptual models of nursing*. Philadelphia: F. A. Davis.

Harvey, W. (1965). *Works: Translation from Latin, with life of the author* (R. Willis, Trans.). New York: Johnson Reprint. (Original work published 1847)

Huch, M. H. (1991). Perspectives on health. *Nursing Science Quarterly, 4*(1), 33-40.

King, I. M. (1971). *Toward a theory for nursing*. New York: John Wiley.

King, I. (1981). *A theory for nursing: Systems, concepts, process*. Albany, NY: Delmar.

King, I. (1990). Health as the goal for nursing. *Nursing Science Quarterly, 3*(3), 123-128.

La Mettrie, J. O. de. (1960). *L'homme machine* (A. Varatanian, Ed.). Princeton, NJ: Princeton University Press. (Original work published 1948)

Magan, S. J. (1987). A critique of King's theory. In R. R. Parse (Ed.), *Nursing science. Major paradigms, theories, and critiques* (pp. 115-133). Philadelphia: W. B. Saunders.

Marriner-Tomey, A. (1989). *Nursing theorists and their work* (2nd ed.). St. Louis, MO: C. V. Mosby.

Meleis, A. (1991). *Theoretical nursing* (2nd ed.). Philadelphia: J. B. Lippincott.

Prigogine, I., & Stengers, I. (1984). *Order out of chaos*. New York: Bantam.

Smith, J. (1983). *The idea of health: Implications for the nursing professional*. New York: Columbia University, Teachers College.

Von Bertalanffy, L. (1952). *Problems of life: An evaluation of modern biological thought*. New York: John Wiley.

Von Bertalanffy, L. (1962). *Modern theories of development: An introduction to theoretical biology* (J. Woodger, Trans.). New York: Harper & Brothers. (Original work published 1933)

Von Bertalanffy, L. (1967). *Robots, men, and minds: Psychology in the modern world*. New York: George Braziller.

Von Bertalanffy, L. (1968a). *General systems theory*. New York: George Braziller.

Von Bertalanffy, L. (1968b). *Organismic psychology and systems theory*. Barre, MA: Clark University Press.

Von Bertalanffy, L. (1976). Introduction. In H. H. Werley, A. Zuzick, M. Zajkowski, & A. D. Zagornik (Eds.), *Health research: The systems approach* (pp. 5-13). New York: Springer.

Von Bertalanffy, L. (1981). *A systems view of man.* Boulder, CO: Westview.

5

Development of a Theory of Departmental Power

CHRISTINA L. SIELOFF

Several disciplines have attempted to define and clarify the construct of power. This process has resulted in multiple definitions of power and a variety of research findings, many of which cannot be combined due to different philosophical bases.

Nursing literature has also discussed the construct of power. However, many publications address nursing's lack of power or nursing's inability to use power that the profession should have (Gonot, 1984). Although a few authors (Maas, 1988; Stuart, 1986) have proposed strategies for nurses and nursing to actualize power, the majority of publications have focused on analyzing the reasons that nurses lack power.

One use for a nursing perspective of power is in nursing administration. Conceptual understanding of power in and for nursing would facilitate research on the power of a nursing department within a health care organization. However, few have attempted to do this with the construct of power (Barrett, 1986; Hawks, 1991). Nurses work with and provide care to people. Nursing needs a perspective of power that addresses this human context of the profession. One way to provide a nursing perspective is to examine the construct from the framework of a nurse theorist (Jennings & Meleis, 1988).

King (1981) identifies the construct of power as relevant to the study of social systems by nurses. In addition, King suggests that work systems of nurses (departmental systems) are appropriate for study by nurses within a social system context.

The purpose of this chapter is to examine the literature on the construct of power and conceptualize the construct within King's (1981) framework. Through reformulation and synthesis, a new theory of departmental system power will be developed. Several research hypotheses generated from the theory will be presented. This will facilitate the development of a knowledge base on power that can then be applied in nursing organizations.

Theory Development Strategies

An analysis of King's (1981) systems framework reveals that she uses a theory development strategy of borrowing and reformulating knowledge from other disciplines (Fitzpatrick & Whall, 1983). Hence, it would be consistent to borrow a theory of power from another discipline and apply it within the social system context of a nursing departmental system (hereafter, nursing department). However, a borrowed theory of power will not reflect the disciplinary perspective of nursing. One way to capture a nursing perspective is to use a nursing conceptual framework through which to filter theories borrowed from other disciplines. Thus, reformulation and synthesis will be used as strategies to develop a nursing theory of power consistent with King's framework.

Reformulation requires that a theory be reconceptualized in terms of nursing and King's (1981) framework. Selected constructs and their relationships from the strategic contingencies' theory of power developed by Hickson, Hinings, Lee, Schneck, and Pennings (1971) will be the basis for reconceptualization.

Following reformulation of constructs from the strategic contingencies' theory, synthesis will then be used to incorporate empirical observations and constructs of King's (1981) framework in the emerging theory of departmental power.

Review of the Literature

Power: Definitions

There are multiple definitions of the construct of power throughout the literature (Douglass & Bevis, 1983; Etzioni, 1975; Katz & Kahn, 1966; Pfeffer, 1981; Yura & Walsh, 1979; Zald, 1970). Such multiple definitions may be due to the abstract nature of power. "Power takes on a very precise meaning only when the analysis is applied to a particular situation, and such application depends on the purposes of the particular analyst concerned" (Astley & Sachdeva, 1984, p. 104).

In her 1981 book, King discussed power, referring to Katz and Kahn (1966), Zald (1970), and Etzioni (1975). In the process of discussing power, she (King, 1981) presents several statements that could be considered definitions of power:

> 1) the process whereby one or more persons influence other persons in a situation, . . . 2) an ability to control events and behaviors in specific situations, . . . 3) the capacity of a person or a group to achieve goals (p. 127), . . . 4) a social force that organizes and maintains society, . . . 5) the ability to use and to mobilize resources to achieve goals, . . . 6) the energy of the organization. (p. 128)

In discussing power in this manner, King inferred that power could be relevant in each of the three systems within her systems framework: personal (Statements 2, 3, 5), interpersonal (Statements 1, 2, 3, 5), and social (Statements 2, 3, 4, 5, 6).

Power: Capacity

The conceptualization of power as a capacity has been supported by many authors (Barrett, 1986; Dawson, 1986; Etzioni, 1970; Maas, 1988; Morriss, 1987; Parsons, 1954). As a capacity, a departmental system's power within a suprasystem would not necessarily depend on the amount of power of other departmental systems as proposed by the idea of zero-based power. Each departmental system would have its own power capacity that could increase without an associated decrease in the capacities of other subsystems. King (1981) also supports the conceptualization of power as a capacity and identifies two components of power: (a) potential power or capacity (Statements 2, 3, 6), and (b) power that is used (Statements 1, 3, 5).

Power as Negative or Positive

Traditionally, in both general and nursing literature, power has had a negative connotation. However, power is not inherently positive or negative; how it is used determines its strengths or deficits (Brown, Gebbie, & Moore, 1978). Other authors also identified that power can be viewed positively (Leininger, 1979; May, 1972; Peterson, 1979; Schrock, 1987).

Power can be seen as positive within King's (1981) framework for several reasons: (a) it is essential for the maintenance of balance and harmony within an organization; (b) it is essential for order in society; and (c) it is used for the achievement of goals.

Power Directions

Generally, three main directions of power are identified in the literature (Beck, 1982). *Vertical power* occurs within superior and subordinate relationships. *Horizontal power* occurs within "relationships between similarly ranked [individuals or] units which differ in function rather than rank" (Dennis, 1983, p. 52). *Subunit power* "is the exertion of power by subunits within an organization to obtain critical resources of the organization for their own department" (Beck, 1982, p. 7). Even with these definitions of power directions delineated, authors often use the terms interchangeably. Such confusion has served to cloud attempts to delineate clearly the direction of power under examination.

The majority of information and research addresses power from the perspective of an individual within a vertical power context. Although this information would prove helpful in analyzing the nurse administrator's power within a health care suprasystem, it provides little assistance in analyzing a departmental system's power within a health care suprasystem.

Sources of Power

Similar to the multiple definitions of power, sources of power are also identified throughout the literature. French and Raven (1959) identified six classical sources of power: (a) reward, (b) punishment, (c) information, (d) legitimate, (e) expert, and (f) referent. Filley and House (1969) reviewed the writings of several authors from 1938 to 1965 and summarized proposed sources of power as (a) control of rewards and sanctions, (b) coercion, (c) legitimacy, (d) expertise, and (e) personal liking.

In the nursing literature, Brown et al. (1978) identified the following sources of power: (a) resources, (b) information, (c) economics, (d) heredity, and (e) charisma. Diers's (1978) power sources included (a) numbers (the size of the nursing group), (b) position power, (c) organized group action, (d) nursing knowledge, and (e) positive thinking. King (1981) identified the following as possible sources of power without elaborating further: (a) resources, (b) position in organization, (c) authority, (d) the role one enacts, (e) goals, (f) environmental forces, and (g) support and respect of others.

The majority of authors addressing sources of power identify these sources from the perspective of an individual within a vertical power context. Although these sources of individual power might be applicable to a group, they cannot automatically be incorporated into a power theory for a group without further examination.

Power and Systems

Within an open system, such as a health care suprasystem, power results from the interdependent relationships between systems or departments within the suprasystem. As a subsystem of a health care suprasystem, each department interacts to maintain the steady state of the suprasystem (Von Bertalanffy, 1968). These interactions reflect the interdependent relationships between departments. All interdependent systems have interdependent relationships between them. Within these interdependent relationships, power is actualized (Finkelstein, 1992; Saunders, 1990). As systems constantly change to maintain a steady state (Von Bertalanffy, 1968), departments also change in their interactions with other departments within a health care suprasystem. The situation determines which system has higher power. Hence, power is not static but changes as situations and interdependencies change.

Power: Strategic Contingencies' Theory

The strategic contingencies' theory of power tries to explain the different amounts of power of different subunits within organizations by focusing on structural power sources. Hickson et al. (1971) states that "when organizations are conceived as interdepartmental systems, the division of labor becomes the ultimate source of intraorganizational power, and power is explained by variables that are elements of each subunit's task, its functioning, and its links with the activities of other subunits" (p. 217).

Hickson, Hinings, Pennings, and Schneck's (1972) research supports three sources of power for a subunit: (a) centrality of work flow, (b) substitutability of activities, and (c) coping with uncertainty. Hickson et al. (1971) define a subunit's *centrality* as the "degree to which its activities are interlinked into the system" (p. 221). Hickson et al. (1971) emphasized the importance of this construct to the analysis of power when stating that "any relationship between coping with uncertainty and power must, in some degree, rest upon the centrality of that coping to the output of the rest of the organization" (p. 75).

Substitutability is defined by Hickson et al. (1971) as the "ability of the organization to obtain alternative performance for the activities of a subunit" (p. 221). They hypothesized that, if a subunit's activities could not be replaced, it would have more power within the organization.

Uncertainty arises from a "lack of information about future events, so that alternatives and their outcomes are unpredictable" (Hickson et al., 1971, p. 219). Hickson et al. (1971) identified coping as a "means to deal with these uncertainties for adequate task performance" (p. 219). Accordingly, it is not the uncertainty that creates power; it is *coping* with the uncertainty that creates power for a subunit. Through its coping, a subunit increases certainty for other subunits by "controlling what are otherwise contingencies for other activities" (Hickson et al., 1972, p. 75). The resulting dependent relationships create power for the coping subunit.

These three variables—centrality, substitutability, and coping with uncertainty—result in power for a subunit because of the involved interdependent relationships. Coping with uncertainty has been found to be the most important factor in determining subunit power. However, the three variables have not been found to function independently but, rather, act in combination to create power for a subunit. Hinings, Hickson, Pennings, and Schneck (1974) identify that a subunit could achieve "first rank power" (p. 40) only through achieving high levels of all three variables.

Power and the Role of the
Leader in Subunit Power

Little direction was available in the literature regarding the role of the group leader in actualizing a subunit's power. The majority of the literature discusses the power of a group leader, not the ability of the leader to actualize group power.

Although not empirically studied, a few authors have presented ideas regarding the role of group leader in the actualization of a group's power. Lips (1981) identified that people in positions of power in organizations must be able to empower others. This idea was supported by Prescott and Dennis (1985) in a study that explored power and powerlessness in nursing departments. The researchers found that "study participants cited the [chief nurse executive] as a critical determinant of nursing department power" (p. 353). As a group leader, a chief nurse executive is seen as important in determining the level of power of the nursing group or department (Blaney, Hobson, & Scodro, 1988).

Group leaders can also negatively affect the power of a group.

> Leaders who are reluctant to exercise the powers inherent in their
> positions can actually undermine the group integrity and thwart
> purposeful achievement. . . . Once staff members sense a leader's
> uncertainty or distaste for wielding power, each "goes his own
> way," group strength dissipates and common projects fail to reach
> their intended goals. (Lapkin, 1986, p. 46F)

A chief nurse executive is seen as a critical subsystem ("subsystem
which carries out certain processes necessary for the system's life"
[Miller, 1969, p. 105]) for a nursing department. This individual
serves as a boundary spanner between the nursing department and
other departments within the health care suprasystem. Without this
individual, the nursing department's interface with other departments would be inconsistent and chaotic. The chief nurse executive
"directs the movement of the [department] toward departmental and
institutional goals" (McFarland & Shiflett, 1979, p. 6).

King (1981) identified that "in the [health care setting], the nurse
brings self to the role" (p. 3). In addition, the nurse also brings
"special knowledge, skills and professional values" (King, 1981, p. 3).
It is proposed that the "self" of a nurse consists of the nurse's special
knowledge, skills, and professional values that relate to the role in
question. On the basis of experiential observations, It is further proposed that the self of the nurse as a chief nurse executive affects the
nursing department's power (Evans, 1989). Therefore, three aspects
of the self of a chief nurse executive that affect the power of a nursing
department are (a) the executive's knowledge of power, (b) the executive's skill in using power, and (c) the value placed on power by the
executive. This conceptualization was supported by King (personal
communication, May 15, 1989).

Defining Departmental System Power

Power: Definition

As identified previously, King (1981) presented six statements,
each of which could be interpreted as a definition of power. The third

statement—"power is the capacity or ability of a person or a group to achieve goals" (King, 1981, p. 127)—has been selected as the basis for defining power because it incorporates aspects of power deemed essential. This definition is positive because it addresses the achievement of goals. The definition allows for a group focus in achieving goals and provides for the consideration of power sources other than resources. Because the definition is being used to define the power of a nursing department, it will be restated as the capacity of a group to achieve goals.

Power: Characteristics

Power as Two Components. Conceptualized as a capacity, power would be present in each nursing department to some degree. However, if all nursing departments have a power capacity, why has a lack of power, also supported in the literature, been observed in many nursing departments? Hence, actualized power is proposed as a second component of the power of a nursing department. This construct (actualized power) has support in the literature. Hickson et al. (1971) spoke of participation or exercised power. King (1981) discussed power that is used separately from power potential.

Power as Positive. Power is identified as a positive strength of a nursing department that can be used by the system to achieve its goals. This use of power to achieve goals has been supported by Etzioni (1970), King (1981), and Hawks (1991).

Direction of Power. The direction of power addressed within this chapter is the power of a departmental system within a health care suprasystem—subunit power. This subunit power would be actualized within situational interactions between the nursing department and other departmental systems within a health care suprasystem as the nursing department seeks to achieve its goals.

Sources of Power. Sources of power identified by King (1981) have been supported in other literature and can also be linked to constructs within the strategic contingencies' theory of power (Hickson et al., 1971). These sources of power, selected for inclusion in the theory, include (a) environmental forces, (b) positions in organizations, (c) roles, (d) resources, and (e) goals.

In summary, departmental system power has (a) two components —a capacity that is universal within all departmental systems and actualized power that results from implementation of the departmental system's power capacity; (b) a positive connotation; (c) a defined direction between subunits; and (d) characteristics within a system— situational, dynamic, goal directed, and occurring within interdependent relationships.

Theory Development

When reformulating a theory from another discipline, the original theory must be examined for congruency with the nursing framework. The strategic contingencies' theory of power (Hickson et al., 1971) has many aspects consistent with King's (1981) framework. Both writings use a systems framework as a basis for theory development. Hickson et al's. (1971) view of organizations as systems of interdependent subunits mutually related in the interdependent activities of a single identifiable social system is consistent with King's (1981) view of a nursing department as a work system of nurses within a health care suprasystem.

Both Hickson et al. (1971) and King (1981) view power as a relevant construct to study within a systems framework. Both also view power as consisting of more than one component and existing within a social or situational relationship. Power, from both perspectives, is located in subunits/systems within organizations/suprasystems, and both approaches address the power of the subunit. Hickson et al.'s (1971) theory focuses on subunits as the units of analysis in addressing power from a subunit viewpoint. King (1981) identified power as "an essential element in social systems" (p. 126) and implied that nursing departments could use power within organizations to achieve goals. She did not, however, address how power between subunits (subsystems) could be increased.

Assumptions

The following assumptions provide a basis for the development of a theory of departmental power:

1. The nursing department is viewed as a departmental system.
2. A nursing department is the focal system of the theory.
3. A nursing department functions within the suprasystem of a health care setting.
4. A critical subsystem of a nursing department is the chief nurse executive.
5. "Power is an essential element in social systems" (King, 1981, p. 126).
6. The subunit power of a nursing department (the power of a nursing department within a health care suprasystem) is the focus of the theory.
7. The total amount of power within a system is not limited.
8. Power has two components, capacity and actualization.
9. Power exists in relation to a situation (King, 1981).
10. Power implies an interdependent relationship (King, 1981).
11. Power resides in positions in organizations (King, 1981).
12. "Power is seen in the role one enacts" (King, 1981, p. 126).

Reconceptualization

The strategic contingencies' theory of power (Hickson et al., 1971) explains power by using subunit variables that are related to the subunit's "task, its functioning, and its links with the activities of other subunits" (Hickson et al., 1971, p. 217). As mentioned previously, three variables (coping with centrality, uncertainty, and substitutability) are identified as critical to the development of subunit power.

King (1981) identifies the following constructs as sources of power within an organization: (a) environmental forces, (b) position, (c) role, (d) resources, and (e) goals. The three primary constructs presented by Hickson et al. (1971) as contributing to a subunit's power within an organization can be reconceptualized as constructs identified by King (1981) as sources of power for a nursing department within a health care suprasystem. Table 5.1 details the linking of variables to construct.

TABLE 5.1 Comparison of Hickson et al's. (1971) and King's (1981) Proposed Sources of Power

Hickson et al. (1971)	King (1981)
Coping with uncertainty	Controlling the effect of environmental forces
Centrality	Position
Substitutability	Role

Environmental forces encountered by a nursing department would create uncertainty for both a nursing department and a health care suprasystem. These forces would originate from the environment within, and external to, a health care suprasystem. These forces would effect not only a nursing department's achievement of goals but also achievement of goals by a health care suprasystem (an event that requires the interdependency of all subsystems within a health care suprasystem).

By controlling the effect of the environmental forces within a health care suprasystem, a nursing department increases its power, which facilitates its achievement of goals. By controlling the effect of the environmental forces, a nursing department also facilitates a health care suprasystem's achievement of goals and, therefore, increases the department's power. As Hickson and his colleagues (1971) identify, it is not the environmental forces that contribute to power, it is the controlling of the effect of those forces that increases the power of a departmental system. Hence, controlling the effect of environmental forces contributes to the level of power of a nursing department.

"Power resides in positions in organizations" (King, 1981, p. 127). The traditional way of identifying the position of a nursing department within a health care suprasystem would be its location on an organizational chart. However, organizational charts identify only the formally prescribed positions within an organization and, frequently, do not indicate the centrality of a department within an organization. Because communication is an important construct within King's framework and the delivery of health care, the position of a nursing department within a health care suprasystem will be defined as the centrality of a nursing department within the communication network of a health care suprasystem. Therefore, the position of a nursing department within a health care suprasystem contributes to the level of power of that nursing department.

"Power is seen in the role one enacts" (King, 1981, p. 126). Within systems, it is expected that departments would function interdependently in the achievement of organizational goals. The role of a nursing department within a health care suprasystem could be defined as the degree to which the work of a health care suprasystem is accomplished through the efforts of a nursing department. It would then be hypothesized that the more pervasive the role of a nursing department within a health care suprasystem, the more difficult it would be to replace the nursing department. Thus, a nursing department's role within a health care suprasystem contributes to the level of power of that nursing department.

In addition to environmental forces, position, and role, King (1981) also identified an additional construct that could effect the power of a nursing department—*resources*. "Power is limited by the resources in a situation" (King, 1981, p. 127). If a departmental system has few resources, it will present as less powerful in a situation in which other departmental systems have more resources. Hence, the resources of a nursing department contribute to the level of power of that nursing department. The resources available to a nursing department may vary by hospital and may include financial resources, personnel, facility space, and so on. The availability of such resources may be dependent on the health care environment. For example, when hospitals focus on generating cost savings related to personnel budgets, unlicensed assistant personnel may be hired in lieu of registered nurses. Hence, in this situation, the departmental resource of the number of registered nurses would decrease.

In summary, a nursing department's power would result from the following variables (as illustrated in Figure 5.1): (a) the ability of a nursing department to control the effect of environmental forces within a health care suprasystem, (b) the position of a nursing department within a health care suprasystem, (c) the role of a nursing department within a health care suprasystem, and (d) the resources available to a nursing department. These variables are proposed to contribute to the first power component of a nursing department— the power capacity of the system.

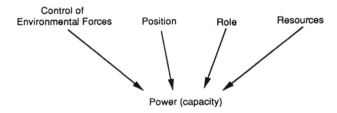

Figure 5.1. Proposed Relationships of Reformulated Constructs With an Additional
          Construct
SOURCE: Evans (1989).

The power capacity of a nursing department is affected by other variables before this capacity can become actualized power. Claus and Bailey (1977) present a conceptualization of power that addresses different aspects of power. These aspects include (a) strength or ability, (b) energy or the willingness to use the ability, and (c) action. It is proposed that a nursing department has power (as a capacity) to achieve its goals as a group. However, the willingness component of departmental power mediates between a nursing department's level of power capacity and its level of actualized power.

Three variables are proposed as willingness or mediating variables between a nursing department's level of power capacity and its level of actualized power. These variables were identified from a review of King's (1981) framework and experiential observations. They are (a) department goals and (b) a chief nurse executive's power ability (see Figure 5.2).

King (1981) states, "The nursing profession cannot use power unless it agrees on a set of unified goals as a basis for group action" (p. 128). This concept, *departmental goals*, was supported in the literature by Schorr (1974).

King (1981) proposed that the personal system can affect both the interpersonal and the social systems. A chief nurse executive (personal system) is proposed as a critical component of a nursing department's (social system) power. The self or personal system of a nurse as a chief nurse executive mediates a nursing department's (social system's) ability to actualize its power capacity. The mediation depends on aspects of self related to the power capacity level of a nursing department: (a) a chief nurse executive's knowledge of power, (b) a chief nurse executive's skill in using power, and (c) the

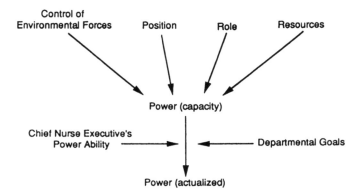

Figure 5.2.   Proposed Relationships of Constructs Contributing to Power Capacity
and Constructs That Mediate the Actualization of Power Capacity
SOURCE: Evans (1989).

importance of power as viewed by a chief nurse executive. These
three aspects combine to compose the chief nurse executive's power
ability (see Figure 5.3).

A nursing department may have a high level of power capacity as
a result of (a) controlling the effect of environmental forces, (b) its
position and role within a health care suprasystem, and (c) its
resources. But, if a nursing department lacks clarity of departmental
goals or if a chief nurse executive lacks knowledge of power, lacks
skill in using power, or does not view power as important, the nursing
department's actualization of its power capacity would be severely
compromised.

In summary, a nursing department's control of the effect of environmental forces, its position and role within a health care suprasystem, and its resources contribute to its power capacity. Before its
power capacity can be actualized, departmental goals must be clear,
and the chief nurse executive must view power as important, and
demonstrate knowledge of power and skill in using power.

Each variable is necessary, but not sufficient, for a nursing department to have a high level of power capacity and to actualize that
capacity to its fullest. Each variable contributes to the overall power
of a nursing department but is dependent on the other variables if a
nursing department is to actualize its power capacity to its optimum.
The optimal actualization of a nursing department's power capacity

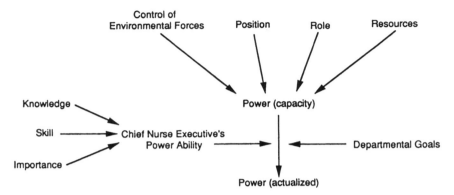

Figure 5.3. Proposed Relationships of the Constructs Within the Theory of Departmental Power
SOURCE: Evans (1989).

will increase the achievement of departmental goals as well as the goals of the broader suprasystem.

Research Hypotheses

As a result of developing the theory of departmental system power, I offer the following propositions from which research questions can be generalized:

1. Controlling the effect of environmental forces, position, resources, and role will be related to nursing department's power capacity.
2. An increase in the nursing department's control of the effect of environmental forces increases the power capacity of that system.
3. An increase in a nursing department's position increases the power capacity of that system.
4. An increase in the role of a nursing department increases the power capacity of that system.
5. An increase in a nursing department's resources increases the power capacity of that system.
6. The existence of clear departmental goals for a nursing department increases the department's actualized power.
7. An increase in a chief nurse executive's knowledge of power will increase the actualized power of a nursing department.

8. An increase in a chief nurse executive's skill in using power will increase the actualized power of a nursing department.

9. An increase in the chief nurse executive's positive view of the importance of power will increase the actualized power of a nursing department.

10. An increase in a nursing department's actualized power will increase the department's achievement of departmental goals.

Summary

Nursing departments need power if they are to achieve departmental goals. Previous literature, although addressing an apparent lack of departmental power, did little to direct departmental actions aimed at increasing power. A theory of departmental system power, derived from King's (1981) systems framework, that can be used to increase a department's power capacity and actualized power has been proposed. Empirical testing of this theory will contribute to the science of nursing in two ways: (a) it will support the validity of King's framework, and (b) it will provide substantive knowledge regarding the power of nursing departments.

References

Astley, W. G., & Sachdeva, P. S. (1984). Structural sources of intraorganizational power: A theoretical synthesis. *Academy of Management Review,* 9(1), 104-113.

Barrett, E. A. M. (1986). Investigation of the principle of helicy: The relationship of human field motion and power. In V. M. Malinski (Ed.), *Explorations on Martha Rogers' science of unitary human beings* (pp. 173-184). Norwalk, CT: Appleton-Century-Crofts.

Beck, C. T. (1982). The conceptualization of power. *Advances in Nursing Science,* 4(2), 1-17.

Blaney, D. R., Hobson, C. J., & Scodro, J. (1988). *Cost effective nursing practice: Guidelines for nurse managers.* Philadelphia: J. B. Lippincott.

Brown, B. J., Gebbie, K., & Moore, J. F. (1978). Affecting nursing goals in health care. *Nursing Administration Quarterly,* 2(3), 17-31.

Claus, K., & Bailey, I. (1977). *Power and influence in health care.* St. Louis, MO: C. V. Mosby.

Dawson, S. (1986). *Analyzing organizations.* London: Macmillan.

Dennis, K. E. (1983). Nursing's power in the organization: What research has shown. *Advances in Nursing Science, 8*(1), 47-57.

Diers, D. (1978). A different kind of energy: Nurse-power. *Nursing Outlook, 26*(1), 51-55.

Douglass, L. M., & Bevis, E. O. (1983). *Nursing management and leadership in action* (4th ed.). St. Louis, MO: C. V. Mosby.

Etzioni, A. (1970). Power as a societal force. In M. E. Olsen (Ed.), *Power in societies* (pp. 18-27). London: Macmillan.

Etzioni, A. (1975). *A comparative analysis of complex organizations: On power, involvement, and their correlates.* New York: Free Press.

Evans, C. L. S. (1989). *Development of a departmental theory of power within Imogene King's framework.* Unpublished manuscript.

Filley, A. C., & House, R. J. (1969). *Managerial process and organizational behavior.* Glenview, IL: Scott, Foresman.

Finkelstein, S. (1992). Power in top management teams: Dimensions, measurement and validation. *Academy of Management Journal, 35*(3), 505-538.

Fitzpatrick, J. J., & Whall, A. L. (1983). *Conceptual models of nursing: Analysis and application.* Bowie, MD: Robert J. Brady.

French, J. R. P., & Raven, B.(1959). The bases of social power. In D. Cartwright (Ed.), *Studies in social power* (pp. 150-167). Ann Arbor: University of Michigan Press.

Gonot, P. J. (1984). *Influence strategies: Impact of organizational variables on patterns of use among hospital-employed nurses.* Unpublished doctoral dissertation, Wayne State University, Detroit, MI.

Hawks, H. H. (1991). Power: A concept analysis. *Journal of Advanced Nursing, 16,* 754-762.

Hickson, D. J., Hinings, C. R., Lee, C. A., Schneck, R. E., & Pennings, J. M. (1971). A strategic contingencies' theory of intraorganizational power. *Administrative Science Quarterly, 16,* 216-229.

Hickson, D. J., Hinings, C. R., Pennings, J. M., & Schneck, R. E. (1972). Contingencies and conditions in intraorganizational power. In A. R. Negandhi, H. Aldrich, G. G. Darkenwald, D. J. Hickson, C. R. Hinings, J. M. Pennings, R. E. Schneck, & L. R. Pondy (Eds.), *Conflict and power in complex organizations: An inter-institutional perspective* (pp. 73-91). Kent, OH: Kent State University Press.

Hinings, C. R., Hickson, D. J., Pennings, J. M., & Schneck, R. E. (1974). Structural conditions of intraorganizational power. *Administrative Science Quarterly, 19*, 22-44.

Jennings, B. M., & Meleis, A. I. (1988). Nursing theory and administrative practice: Agenda for the 1990s. *Advances in Nursing Science, 10*(3), 56-69.

Katz, D., & Kahn, R. L. (1966). *The social psychology of organization.* New York: John Wiley.

King, I. M. (1981). *A theory for nursing: Systems, concepts, process.* New York: John Wiley.

Leininger, M. M. (1979). Territoriality, power and creative leadership in administrative nursing contexts. *Nursing Dimensions, 7*(2), 33-42.

Lips, H. M. (1981). *Women, men, & the psychology of power.* Englewood Cliffs, NJ: Prentice Hall.

Maas, M. L. (1988). A model of organizational power: Analysis and significance to nursing. *Research in Nursing and Health, 11*, 153-163.

May, R. (1972). *Power and innocence: A search for the source of violence.* New York: Norton.

McFarland, D. E., & Shiflett, N. (1979). The role of power in the nursing profession. *Nursing Dimensions, 7*(2), 1-13.

Miller, J. (1969). Living systems: Basic concepts. In W. Gray, F. J. Duhl, & N. D. Rizzo (Eds.), *General systems theory and psychiatry* (pp. 51-133). Boston: Little, Brown.

Morriss, P. (1987). *Power: A philosophical analysis.* Manchester, England: Manchester University Press.

Parsons, T. (1954). *Essays in sociological theory* (rev. ed.). New York: Free Press.

Peterson, G. G. (1979). Power: A perspective for the nurse administrator. *Journal of Nursing Administration, 9*(7), 7-10.

Pfeffer, J. (1981). *Power in organizations.* Cambridge, MA: Ballinger.

Prescott, P. A., & Dennis, K. E. (1985). Power and powerlessness in hospital nursing departments. *Journal of Professional Nursing, 1*(6), 348-355.

Saunders, C. S. (1990). The strategic contingencies' theory of power: Multiple perspectives. *Journal of Management Studies, 27*(1), 1-18.

Schorr, T. M. (1974). Nurse power. *American Journal of Nursing, 74*(6), 1047.

Schrock, R. A. (1987). Professionalism—A critical examination. In L. Hockey (Ed.), *Recent advances in nursing* (pp. 12-24). Singapore: Longman.

Stuart, G. W. (1986). An organizational strategy for empowering nursing. *Nursing Economic$, 4*(2), 69-73.

Von Bertalanffy, L. (1968). *General systems theory: Foundation, development, applications.* New York: George Braziller.

Yura, H., & Walsh, M. (1979). Concepts and theories related to leadership. *Nursing Dimensions, 7*(2), 75-86.

Zald, M. N. (1970). *Power in organizations.* Nashville, TN: Vanderbilt University Press.

—— 6 ——

King's Interacting
Systems and Empathy

MARTHA RAILE ALLIGOOD

GINGER W. EVANS

DOROTHY L. WILT

In this chapter, the nursing phenomenon, empathy, will be viewed from the perspective of King's (1981) interacting systems. Empathy is a prominent theme in nursing literature. Most nursing textbooks, such as those for psychiatric nursing, medical-surgical nursing, and pediatric nursing, which cover psychosocial aspects of nursing, include a section on empathy. Furthermore, empathy has become a popular strategy used to market programs of hospitals, nursing homes, and other health care agencies (Brenner et al., 1986). In contrast to the prominence of empathy in nursing textbooks and promotional materials, the empathy research literature has pointed out theoretical and methodological problems in empathy studies (Alligood, 1992). Among the problems identified in nursing empathy studies, a major one is the varied definitions used in conceptual frameworks from other disciplines as well as their tools of measurement (Gagan, 1983). For example, *Webster's New Universal Unabridged Dictionary* (1992) defines empathy in two ways:

> empathy: 1. the intellectual identification with or vicarious experiencing of the feelings, thoughts, or attitudes of another. 2. the imaginative ascribing to an object, as a natural object or work of art, feelings or attitudes present in oneself. (p. 482)

This chapter conceptualizes the nursing phenomenon of empathy in King's (1981) interacting systems framework and describes its nature in nursing.

Clearly, empathy is a nursing phenomenon and needs to be studied from a nursing perspective. King's (1981) framework of interacting systems lends itself to studies of the interactive complexity of this nursing phenomenon because each system addresses the impact of the empathic process and is, therefore, the framework of choice. King's (1971, 1981) conceptual framework has three systems that articulate with one another: the personal system, interpersonal system, and social system. Initially, empathy will be defined with a working definition that will be further developed in each of King's interacting systems. Empathy is conceptualized as a developmental phenomenon (Alligood, 1992; Smither, 1977). King's interacting systems are used as a guide for understanding the development of empathy in nursing students. Throughout this chapter, the development of empathy in nursing will be presented in the context of nursing students because nurses' learning of how to use their own empathy begins here.

Empathy is a key ingredient in each of King's (1981) three systems because, as a feeling attribute of persons (Alligood, 1992), it is the manner by which the nurse learns to recognize and respond intrapersonally to nursing situations (personal system). This can be seen by a review of the personal system concepts that King has included.

Personal System

The personal system concepts include (a) perception, (b) self, (c) growth and development, (d) body image, (e) time, and (f) space (King, 1981, p. 19).

Perception

Perception is defined as "a process of organizing, interpreting, and transforming information from sense data and memory. It is a process of human transactions with environment. It gives meaning to one's experience, represents one's image of reality, and influences one's behavior" (King, 1981, p. 24). King makes application of perception to nursing and points out that perception is influenced by emotion. She further emphasizes the importance of perceptual accuracy (King, 1981). If perceptual accuracy is affected by emotion, then students' understanding of their own emotions influences the way they organize and interpret sense data. Based on King's ideas, empathy is proposed as a dimension of sensory perception. Empathy organizes sense data into a meaningful understanding. Therefore, with empathy, there is not only affective knowing but also an interpretation of what is known. For example, the new mastectomy client who tells her nurse she is "OK, just tired" when asked how she feels gives a verbal response. The nurse hears the words but also hears the low tone of voice and slowed speech pattern. The nurse sees that the client is slumped in posture and disheveled in appearance. The nurse's sense data, organized with empathy, would perceive that this client has just experienced a loss and her behavior is that of sadness. From this perception, accurate goals could be addressed. However, if the nurse organized the sense data by hearing the response "OK, just tired" and, seeing the behavior, concluded that the client is tired postoperatively, a different and possibly less accurate goal would be addressed.

Self

King next addresses the concept of self. "Knowledge of self is a key to understanding human behavior, because self is the way I define me to myself and to others. Self is all that I am" (King, 1981, p. 26). "Awareness of self helps one to become a sensitive human being who is comfortable with self and with relationships with others" (King, 1981, p. 28). We contend that empathy is the affective dimension of human sensitivity that King describes. Through empathy, persons perceive others and they experience an awareness of the situation of the other in themselves (Holden, 1990). This is supported by King's notion that the "self is an open system" (King, 1981, p. 27). Therefore, through empathy, a wide range of human sensitivity is developed, increasing a nurse's use of self. "A concept of self is reflected in patterns of growth and development and in the structure and function of human beings" (King, 1981, p. 28).

Growth and Development

"The manner in which a person grows and develops is influenced positively and negatively by other people and objects in the environment" (King, 1981, pp. 30-31). This being true, student nurses bring to the education experience a history of positive and negative interaction with other people and the environment (Smither, 1977). What we are describing here is developmental empathy that has been a part of a person's life since birth. Not only has it had an impact in the past, but it also influences students' ability to become more sensitive human beings. Growth of this developmental empathy in students is an affective component of what is often described as a cognitive process. For example, early in their education, student nurses are introduced to the concept of empathy, which can influence their cognitive knowing about empathy. However, a nurse educator must also bring students to an experiential understanding of their affective sensing of empathy within the self in preparation for their interpersonal relationships with clients.

Body Image

"Body image is defined as a person's perceptions of his [or her] own body, others' reactions to his [or her] appearance, and is a result of others' reactions to self" (King, 1981, p. 33). The concept of body image relies heavily on empathy because the reaction of others, which may be positive or negative, occurs as people see others reacting to them. "If a client perceives that a body image may limit the ability to achieve a goal, whether or not this is true, a nurse needs to recognize this perception as real and work with the client in order to provide additional feedback" (Evans, 1991, p. 10). Empathy is vital to this circular feedback process, which begins with the initial reac-

tion and facilitates the development of shared respect. As the interaction continues, with bodily changes and additional input, the
perception of body image emerges. Therefore, this dynamic process
is vital to the development of mutual goals.

Time

King (1981) says the following about time: "Time gives unity to
large areas of one's experience. . . . Time is a term used by individuals to give order to events and to determine duration based on
perceptions of each person's experiences" (p. 45). These ideas emphasize the importance of viewing clients in an expanse of time to
increase our understanding of their behavior. Within this context of
time, the otherwise isolated observations of behavior become meaningful to a nurse or student nurse as empathy facilitates a mutual
understanding of those events or behaviors from a scenario in a
patient's life. This interpretation of time in the nurse-patient interaction is supported by King's notion that time is subjective (King,
1981, p. 44). We contend that King's idea of time's being subjective,
or relative to people's perceptions of events in their lives, actually
occurs through the empathetic process. "Spatial-temporal dimensions of the environment influence perceptions, self, body image, and
growth and development" (King, 1981, p. 47). The complexity of the
concept of time in relationship to the other personal system concepts
helps us understand how difficult it is to set mutual goals.

Space

King (1981) sets forth space as an essential component of the
personal system because of its relationship to perception and body
image. "Space is defined as existing in all directions and is the same
everywhere" (King, 1981, p. 37). On the basis of King's premise, we
suggest that space also affects the self. Therefore, all of the linkages
of empathy to King's personal concepts presented so far in this
chapter support the relationship of empathy to space in the personal
system. We suggest that a nurse or student nurse senses the positive
aspects of persons in space as well as the cues of violations of personal
space through empathic knowing. King's (1981) idea that "use of

space and defense of space is nonverbal communication" (p. 38) supports our interpretation of the role of empathy in space.

In summary, these personal system concepts (perception, self, body image, growth and development, space, and time) form a structure for considering personal development, including intrapersonal development. We suggest that empathy is the medium for intrapersonal development of the personal systems of student nurses, which affects the self through perception and body image, resulting in growth and development in time and space. Furthermore, the level of development of students' personal systems is reflected in their interpersonal processes. This leads to the second system in King's conceptual model.

Interpersonal System

The interpersonal system concepts include (a) interaction, (b) communication, (c) transaction, (d) role, and (e) stress (King, 1981, p. 59). The interpersonal concepts form a structure for considering the interaction of personal systems in the interpersonal process of a nurse-patient relationship. In other words, student nurses' personal development affects their capacity to participate in nurse-patient interactions. Therefore, because empathy was found to be vital in student nurses' personal development, it is also reflected in their interpersonal development. This can be seen by reviewing the concepts King includes in the interpersonal system.

Interaction

Although King (1971, 1981) does not discuss empathy per se, her discussions of the "process of interactions between individuals as a sequence of verbal and nonverbal behaviors" (1981, p. 60) may be likened to empathic interaction. For example, her discussion of perception as a sequence of the behaviors of interacting persons, which includes mental action and physical action, is comparable to cognition and psychomotor activity. Although an affective component of this process is absent from King's discussion, we believe development in this area has the capacity to extend King's work. This being true, the phenomenon of empathy logically completes the circle by adding this affective dimension of the component to the cognitive and psychomotor components already included in the interpersonal process.

Communication

From the general systems idea of feedback, it is understood that systems develop ways to send and receive information. Furthermore, information exchange is essential to systems and the effectiveness of communication determines the organization of the system (Anderson & Carter, 1974, p. 27). King's (1981) interacting systems are presented as "systems in process" as set forth by Von Bertalanffy (1968) in *General System Theory*. Empathy is described as a process of interaction that is verbal and nonverbal. Therefore, through the systems idea of feedback, the nursing phenomenon of empathy can be understood as a component of communication in King's systems framework. King (1981) calls for nurses to become aware of the use of nonverbal communication in nursing:

> All human activities that link person to person and person to environment are forms of communication. . . . in most person-oriented professions, such as nursing, knowledge and skills in communication are an important part of professional work as communication forms the basis for interactions with individuals who may be experiencing unusual stress that causes them to seek professional assistance. (p. 79)

Therefore, we propose that empathy is a major component of communication, which is important to the nurse-patient relationship. That is, empathy is the medium whereby the mutual understanding occurs. Empathy has been reported to increase the speed (time) and effectiveness of communication (Kramer & Schmalenberg, 1977).

Transaction

Optimal communication facilitates transactions that, according to King, are the "transfer of value between two or more persons" (1981, p. 81). The ability to be empathetic is consistent with the ability to identify and respect the value of self and others. It is dependent on adequate boundary formation that allows the individual to stand apart from another, caring about one's own values and that of the other person. This has been identified as a vital dimension frequently discussed by others when distinguishing empathy from sympathy (Davis, 1990; Holden, 1990). King (1981) states, "When transactions are made, tension or stress is reduced in a situation" (p. 82). We propose that when patients (or individuals) feel understood and their values are respected empathically, anxiety and tension decrease. This suggests that empathy is a key component in transaction.

Role

Empathy is recognized as a strong component of the nursing role (Holden, 1990). "Role of a nurse," according to King (1981), "can be defined as an interaction between one or more individuals who come to a nursing situation in which nurses perform functions of professional nursing based on knowledge skills and values identified as nursing" (p. 93). In addition, empathy is recognized for its market value within the health care delivery system (Brenner et al., 1986). When patients experience empathy in nurses in the health care delivery system, they value the role of the nurse. Therefore, empathy influences the definition of the role of the nurse. The congruence of role and transaction reduces stress (King, 1981).

Stress

King (1981) describes stress as the final concept of the interpersonal system. She writes, "Nurses are in a position to observe for patterns of behavioral response to stressors and stressful events" (p. 102). As an energy response, stress provides strong cuing for the empathetic nurse who recognizes, as King says, that "stress is negative and positive; it is constructive and destructive" (p. 98). In addition to the cognitive understanding of a patient's stress, empathetic perception organizes the input to form a deeper, more meaningful knowledge of the patient's experience, thereby facilitating the mutual goal setting and coping strategies to accomplish goal attainment. This is also noted by Rawnsley (1980), who suggests that

empathy facilitates coordination with another's goal attainment
(p. 243). "Once [stressors are] identified, nurses are in a position to
take some action to decrease, reduce, or eliminate some factors that
produce stress" (King, 1981, p. 102). This is accomplished through
the mutual process outlined by King (1981) in her interpersonal
system and, more explicitly, in her theory of goal attainment, which
she has derived from selected personal and interpersonal system
concepts. The level of development of the personal and the interpersonal systems of nursing students is reflected by their performance
in the larger social system.

Social System

The final system in King's (1981) conceptual framework is the
social system. The social system concepts include (a) organization,
(b) authority, (c) power, (d) status, and (e) decision making (p. 114).
The social system provides a context for consideration of the intrapersonal development of nursing students, which manifests itself
in their interpersonal processes with patients, instructors, and other
students. Within this context, students are led to an understanding
of the interrelationship of their personal and interpersonal processes
as they progress through their nursing education. The development
that occurs through this educational process leads students toward
professional development that is best understood in the context of
King's social system. Therefore, this development will be discussed
from the perspective of King's social system concepts.

Organization

"An organization is a system whose continuous activities are
conducted to achieve goals. In this system of activities, the roles of
individuals depict the human elements of complex interrelated systems in organizations" (King, 1981, p. 119). For example, student
nurses are part of a preliminary organization that is a college or
university for education. The goal of nursing education is to transmit
knowledge that prepares an individual for level of entry into the
nursing profession and the ability to deliver initial, quality, compe-

tent care. When empathy is a qualifier of care that is modeled and taught, the expected outcome is a professional who can achieve standards. According to King (1981), "If nurses are to perform their functions as professionals, they must influence the organization to achieve standards whereby quality care can be measured" (p. 121).

Authority

King (1981) defines authority as

> a transactional process characterized by active, reciprocal relations in which members' values, background, and perception play a role in defining, validating, and accepting the authority of individuals within an organization. One person influences another, and he [or she] recognizes, accepts, and complies with the authority of that person. (p. 124)

Building on the role of empathy in the personal and interpersonal systems discussed earlier, King sets forth authority as a transactional process using lines of authority and channels of formal and informal communication. In other words, for people to function with authority in social systems, they use their empathic development in the personal and interpersonal systems. For example, student nurses being supervised in a clinical area will function and learn more effectively if in their empathic development they have an understanding of the value of authority. Learning is optimal when authority is reciprocal— that is, as the faculty uses empathy to perceive the values and backgrounds of individual students.

Power

Power is defined by King (1981) as "the process whereby one or more persons influence other persons in a situation" (p. 127). Similar to authority, power is also dependent on the empathic process. For example, King's idea of influence relies on human interaction through which words, thoughts, and feelings are shared and decisions are made. Student nurses are empowered through this developmental process, drawing on their personal and interpersonal life experiences to function with power and authority in making nursing decisions at this social system level. Even as students, nurses are able to influence goal attainment. King (1981) has postulated that "power is directly related to authority" (p. 127). Therefore, the students' use of power and authority leads to their status.

Status

Status is defined by King as the "position of an individual in a group or a group in relation to other groups in an organization" (King, 1981, p. 129). King further specifies status as situational. As mentioned earlier, the educational system is their organization while students are learning. Therefore, the status of nursing students is dependent on their power and authority in that organization. Through the educational organization, students develop their empathic abilities at the personal, interpersonal, and, finally, social system levels. This empathic development is critical to student nurses' sense of status and their decision-making abilities.

Decision Making

King (1981) defines decision making as "a dynamic and systematic process by which goal-directed choice of perceived alternatives is made and acted upon by individuals or groups to answer a question and attain a goal" (p. 132). Empathy contributes to decision making via the dynamic process, the perception of alternatives, and the sensitivity with which a nurse takes action. Decision making is at the heart of nursing practice because through the decision-making process, the nurse brings to fruition personal and interpersonal capacities.

The delivery of safe, effective nursing care is dependent on an understanding of self and others in the context of the profession. Empathy is proposed as a nursing phenomenon that is a way of knowing for a nurse and that facilitates system development in all three of King's interacting systems. In the interpersonal system, empathy is a vital aspect of the communication process between persons as they feel the situation, whether in the nurse-patient relationship (Bergman, 1983) or in the student-instructor relationship (Rosendahl, 1973). Finally, a student learns to practice nursing appropriately in the context of the nursing profession. In the social system, empathy is key because each nurse's ongoing development as a nurse is dependent on the capacity to be appropriate, effective, and influential and also see the self in relation to the task at hand (nursing) personally, interpersonally, and professionally.

King's (1981) systems framework of three interacting systems provides a structure for understanding the development of empathy at each system level and from which to pose propositions of the interrelationships of these systems that can then be tested in research. The quality of such studies is dependent on a conceptual structure that provides a view of phenomena of concern to nursing. King's interacting systems form a basis for the consideration and study of the phenomenon of empathy.

Furthermore, conceptualizing empathy in King's (1981) systems framework bypasses the problems experienced in nursing and other disciplines about the objective and subjective perspectives. Empathy in systems need not be objective or subjective because it is integrated (Holden, 1990). This integrated process provides the foundation for understanding empathy as a developmental phenomenon. King's interacting systems framework guided this process in articulating the description of this human feeling attribute.

This conceptualization of empathy in King's work also has implications for clarifying the nature of the definition of empathy for nursing. As noted earlier, a dictionary defines empathy in two ways, separating the intellectual from the artistic form. The analysis reported in this chapter suggests a blending of the two in process, leading to an understanding of empathy in nursing that moves beyond separation of science and art (Rhodes, 1990).

In summary, this chapter has introduced the nursing phenomena of empathy in King's (1981) interactive systems framework. Using the concepts that King includes in each system as a structure for the chapter, empathy has been proposed as a vital dimension of the dynamic human interactive process of each system. King's (1981) interacting systems framework is proposed as a structure for researchers to pose propositions for study of the phenomenon of empathy. Finally, the implications of this chapter for clarifying the definition of empathy in the discipline of nursing are addressed.

References

Alligood, M. (1992). Empathy: The importance of recognizing two types. *Journal of Psychosocial Nursing, 30*(3), 14-17.

Anderson, R., & Carter, I. (1974). *Human behavior in a social environment.* Chicago: Aldine.

Bergman, R. (1983). Understanding the patient in all his human needs. *Journal of Advanced Nursing, 8,* 185-190.

Brenner, P., Boyd, D., Thompson, T., Marz, M., Buerhaus, P., & Leininger, M. (1986). The care symposium: Considerations for nursing administrators. *Journal of Nursing Administration, 16*(1), 25-30.

Davis, C. (1990). What is empathy, and can empathy be taught? *Physical Therapy, 70*(11), 707-715.

Evans, C. (1991). *Imogene King: A conceptual framework for nursing.* Newbury Park, CA: Sage.

Gagan, J. (1983). Methodological notes on empathy. *Advances in Nursing Science, 5*(2), 65-72.

Holden, R. (1990). Empathy: The art of emotional knowing in holistic nursing care. *Holistic Nursing Practice, 5*(1), 70-79.

King, I. (1971). *Toward a theory of nursing.* New York: John Wiley.

King, I. (1981). *A theory of goal attainment.* New York: John Wiley.

Kramer, M., & Schmalenberg, C. (1977). The first job-approving ground: Basis for empathy development. *Journal of Nursing Administration, 7*(1), 12-20.

Rawnsley, M. (1980). Toward a conceptual base for affective nursing. *Nursing Outlook, 28*(4), 244-247.

Rhodes, J. (1990). *A philosophical study of the art of nursing explored within a metatheoretical framework of philosophy of art and aesthetics.* Unpublished doctoral dissertation, University of South Carolina, Columbia.

Rosendahl, P. (1973). Effectiveness of empathy, non-possessive warmth, and genuineness of self-actualization of nursing students. *Nursing Research, 22*(3), 252-257.

Smither, S. (1977). A reconsideration of the developmental study of empathy. *Human Development, 20,* 253-276.

Von Bertalanffy, L. (1968). *General system theory.* New York: George Braziller.

Webster's new universal unabridged dictionary. (1992). New York: Barnes & Noble.

7

The Concept of Space in King's Systems Framework

Its Implications for Nursing

LISELOTTE ROOKE

The discipline of nursing is evolving, and nursing conceptual models are seen as useful ways to develop the discipline. When a discipline is developing, there is a demand for the use of conceptual models and theories of different levels of abstraction that emerge from the core of the discipline. Connected to the striving to promote a discipline is an interest in legitimating the profession. One main criterion for a profession, according to Greenwood (1957), is that systematic theories exist that develop from the practice of the profession. As a result, the discipline of nursing is challenged to improve professional nursing practice by using nursing conceptual models and theories. This includes further developing and refining existing nursing conceptual models and generating hypotheses from them.

Explicating the Purpose of the Study

There has been debate about the difficulties of testing nursing theories and evaluating conceptual models of nursing. A main theme in the debate has been the lack of clarity in what is meant by theory testing (Acton, Irvin, & Hopkins, 1991; Silva, 1986; Silva & Rothart, 1984; Silva & Sorrell, 1992). One purpose of this study is to challenge some of these difficulties and to demonstrate an inductive way of evaluating a concept in a nursing conceptual model—in this case, the concept of space in King's (1981) systems framework.

King's (1981) framework consists of three systems: the personal system, the interpersonal system, and the social system. In each system, there are interrelated concepts, which together describe important aspects of nursing. The personal system includes seven concepts: (a) perception, (b) self, (c) growth and development, (d) body image, (e) space, and (f) time, all of which have implications for nursing practice. In 1986, King added one more concept to the personal system: (g) the concept of learning. This study is focused on the concept of space and its implications for nursing.

A major need for nursing research, according to Whall (1989), is to examine specific concepts in the existing conceptual models of nursing. Interest in this study emerged from nurses working in nursing homes who attended a course on nursing models. The nurses found King's systems framework particularly useful. They decided to study the concept of space more thoroughly. They considered that the concept of space would give new dimensions to their understanding of nursing practice (Rooke, 1990). This study can be seen as a way to describe the concept of space in King's framework and to give it a practical dimension.

The Concept of Space

The concept of space is relevant for many disciplines: for example, anthropology, architecture, ethnology, psychology, sociology, and nursing. As a consequence of this, space is defined in different ways. Altman (1975) points out, however, that the different definitions often have the common theme of ownership of a place. Bakker and

Bakker-Rabdau (1973) define space as the area of an individual's life experienced as one's own, in which he or she has control, takes initiative, has expertise, or accepts responsibility. Hall (1966) says that an individual's sense of space is related to self-awareness, which is in a near interaction with the environment. Hall describes how the individual has a special sense of distance, which is related to the comprehension of space. Hall distinguishes between four distances:

- Intimate distance (close phase and far phase, 0-18 inches)
- Personal distance (close phase and far phase, 1.5-4 feet)
- Social distance (close phase and far phase, 4-12 feet)
- Public distance (close phase and far phase, 12 feet and more)

According to Hall (1966), the intimate space can be regarded as the space where the person gives love, care, and protection. Even actions of a more aggressive nature, such as fighting and wrestling, are characteristic of the intimate space. The personal space is often defined as an "invisible bubble," an area immediately around the body. In this space, the voice is normal, in contrast to the intimate space, where the voice is often lower. The social space is often seen at work, where individuals tend to mark off their social space, for instance, with their own writing table, own room, and so on. In the social space, the voice is often higher than normal.

Personal and social distances should not be regarded as constant phenomena, because they fluctuate a great deal due to the situation and the interpersonal relationship between the involved persons. Altman (1975) proposes that the personal space is affected by individual factors, interpersonal factors, and situational factors. People tend to avoid intrusion of their space and may feel distress or embarrassment if avoidance is not possible.

The public distance can be seen in more official situations—for example, when a person gives a speech at a banquet. The public distance has no relevance for direct nursing care and is therefore not used in the study.

When using a concept that is of interest to more than one discipline, it is important to assimilate the concept into the discipline in question. Both the concept and the discipline might benefit from each other in a dialectical way. King (1981) defines space as "the physical area called territory and by the behavior of individuals occupying space. . . . Personal space is related to time, distance, area, volume, perception, and communication" (p. 38). King's definition stresses, as does Altman's (1975), the need of ownership of a space. King (1981) also relates the concept of space to three other concepts in her framework: time, perception, and communication. In regard to the scientific development of a discipline, it is important to describe and specify salient concepts for the discipline in question. King's framework can be regarded as an important contribution to the nursing discipline for this purpose.

Method

The method in this study is based on the critical incident method (Flanagan, 1949, 1954). Also, Benner (1984) has provided inspiration for the study. Benner identifies the importance of elucidating nursing knowledge embedded in practice by using the critical incident method, through nurses relating nursing stories in a narrative way.

Seven experienced nurses who attended a course on nursing conceptual models as a part of a research project described critical situations related to the concept of space (Rooke, 1990). The written situations came from their daily practice at a geriatric hospital. To reach saturation, according to the number of related situations, other experienced nurses and nursing educators who attended other courses on conceptual models were asked to describe critical situations that could be related to concepts in King's systems framework. These nurses came from specialties such as medical nursing, surgical nursing, geriatrics, and intensive care.

Narrative Examples in
Relation to the Concept of Space

The narratives related by the nurses and nursing educators in the different courses are categorized by means of Hall's (1966) distances: the intimate space, the personal space, and the social space. This system of space categories can be related to King's (1981) view of space. The nursing situations demonstrate that space has a meaningful dimension for nursing care. Some situations show in a reversed way that an important aspect of nursing care is respecting an individual's space. Clearly, in some situations the space of the patient was threatened.

Examples Related to Intimate Space

The nurses from the nursing home often described difficulties when they helped demented patients with personal care. The patients often became aggressive because they did not understand the purpose of washing. The following examples illustrate this.

Example 1

Today I came more close to a patient, and I felt good. The patient is demented, she never says anything, maybe "no" sometimes. After all she has her intimate space preserved. . . . She seems to have suffered a lot when we washed her, fed her, combed her hair, changed her diapers. However, she seems sometimes to appreciate what we are doing. Today, when I was washing her, I got a "Thank you," instead of "No, no, no."

Example 2

This is happening every day. You are going to help a patient with washing, dressing. You talk and coax in different ways, but still the patient tries to scratch, pinch and kick you.

Even young patients and patients who are not demented experienced a threat against their intimate space, especially when the staff had to help with personal care. One nurse related the following incident.

Example 3

This is a young woman. She had got multiple fractures after a car accident. She cannot move her legs and her left arm. Due to the high risk for infection, she has high doses of penicillin IV. As secondary effects of the penicillin, she has got frequent diarrhea. When the diarrhea comes, she has to be helped by three nurses.

In these situations, she reacts with irritation and aggressiveness against the nurses.

In the last example, there can be seen a connection between the concept of body image and the concept of space. The young woman may experience being out of control regarding her body. Gonot (1989) proposes a relationship between the concept of space and the concept of body image. It is also possible that the young woman was ashamed of not being able to handle the situation by herself and in that way felt a threat against privacy. This latter possibility highlights Bakker and Bakker-Rabdau's (1973) statement that privacy and security are such important aspects of space that the individual "will spend enormous amounts of time and energy establishing a claim on privacy and defending it against intruders" (p. 4). In the preceding situation, the young woman may have been trying to defend her privacy.

These examples illustrate that patients who cannot control the distance between themselves and the staff may experience threats to their intimate territory. Barron (1990) emphasized, in a study of the patient's personal space, that nurses must preserve the dignity of the patient, for example, when assisting with personal care. The experience of one nurse offered these same thoughts:

> I find patients who are being helped with washing lying totally naked without any screens, or sitting on the toilet with the door wide open, or closed toilet doors are rapidly pushed open, staff are entering without knocking, moving personal belongings without asking, lifting blankets from the patient's bed, sitting down on the patient's bed without asking.

How a person experiences space depends on the relationship between the involved actors (Bakker & Bakker-Rabdau, 1973; Hall, 1966; King, 1981). One nurse at a nursing home with elderly patients regarded space as connected with feelings. She explained that elderly people have a need for some sign of love, such as a hug. But elderly people also have a need to give love to another person. Giving signs of love is connected with letting another person come into one's intimate space. When you give the other person a hug, he or she becomes a part of your own space. The nurse related the following incident.

Example 4

> I had an elderly demented male patient. All the time I had the feeling that he had a need for love and that he wanted to give love back. Therefore, every morning I kissed him on his cheek after his shaving and told him how nice he looked. But he never showed any sign of liking it. . . . But, one day he came up to me and gave me a kiss on my cheek.

Examples Related to Personal Space

The situations that were categorized to illustrate personal space were often connected to interaction between patient and nurse. King (1981) says that interactions are reciprocal, wherein meanings, feelings, and goals are explored. In the two following narratives, related by the same nurse, both the reciprocal action and the effects of a nonreciprocal action can be seen.

Example 1

> One day I heard that one of the elderly female demented patients was shouting from her room. I went into her room and up to her bed without saying anything. I just stood there. After a while I asked her if I could take the chair and sit down. "Yes," she answered. After a moment, she raised her hand, which she had kept under the quilt. She gave me her hand, and we were just sitting like that, until she calmed down.

In this example, the nurse interacted in a way that resulted in the elderly patient's accepting the nurse's entering her personal space. In the next situation, the nurse did not succeed in interacting in the same way and, therefore, she did not reciprocally enter into the patient's personal space.

Example 2

> There was an elderly demented female patient. Her speech was completely incoherent. Sometimes she made up her own words, and sometimes she could say "Yes" and "No" adequately. The woman was sitting in her room with a table in front of her and she was playing with some toy models. I asked, if I could sit down for a while. "Yes," she answered. I tried to talk to her. But she only answered with her incoherent words. I felt the situation becoming

more and more frustrating, and I got a feeling of not being present, so at last I asked her, if she thought I should go away. "Yes," she answered.

The nurse's interpretation of both situations was that the patient answered logically both times. The first time, the nurse was allowed to sit down. The second time the nurse was told to go away, possibly because she did not succeed in building up a situation of trust and understanding between herself and the patient. The interpretations can be related to the concept of space. In the first situation, the patient did not experience a threat against her space. However, in the second situation, the patient might have experienced a breach of her personal space because the nurse did not manage to establish a warm atmosphere. Of course, there is also the possibility that the patient was tired and really wanted the nurse to leave.

The two related situations (Examples 1 and 2) also show a relationship between the concepts of space, interaction, and transaction. In Example 1, transaction occurred and the demented patient calmed down, which may be seen as a mutual goal for patient and nurse. In Example 2, it was the nurse only who had a goal—namely, to talk with the patient and to establish a relationship. If there exists no reciprocity and mutuality in the interaction, transactions are unlikely to occur. In the second example, restriction of personal space interfered with interaction and therefore with transactions and goal attainment. Altman (1975) proposed that space is affected by factors such as interpersonal interactions.

Personal space is connected to the integrity of the individual. One nurse described the following situation, which shows how nurses can threaten personal space. There was an older man with Parkinson's disease, and he often forgot things. The reason he was admitted to the hospital was that he had fallen at home and had injured his right ear. The man had some difficulties in walking.

Example 3

It was early in the morning and we had a staff shortage, so the atmosphere in the ward was tense. We entered the room, where the old man was still asleep. We went up to the window, pulled back the drapes, and woke the old man up and told him that it

was time to get up. We tried to help him because we knew he had
fallen at home. He said impatiently "I can manage myself." When
he was going to wash at the washstand, I took a chair and put it
behind him. The old man said angrily, "I always stand up, when
I wash." He took the chair and threw it against us.

This situation illustrates how space can be connected to integrity
and self-respect. In situations in which the self-respect of individuals
is threatened, they often strive to increase their space in different
ways (Hollmerus-Nilsson, 1985). The man in this situation tried to
increase his space in his own particular way. The interpretation of
the situation may be more simply related to the abrupt awakening.
However, the nurse experienced the behavior as a space-related
behavior.

There were also narratives that illustrated how demented patients
marked their space with different belongings. Bakker and Bakker-
Rabdau (1973) propose that one main territorial behavior is "marking
of an area to indicate ownership" (p. 3). As for demented patients,
this territorial behavior can be rather peculiar, such as marking one's
space by arranging bed lamps or flowers in a special way.

Personal belongings can give some safety to a patient and give a
sense of "This is my space" as illustrated by the following example
given by a nurse at a nursing home. The patient was a distinguished
looking older woman. She lived in a room with three other patients.
The others were demented, but she was not. The nurse often talked
to the patient. One day, the patient told her the following.

Example 4

I take my pillow and my blanket which I have brought from my
home. Then I feel a little like being home, and when the staff
switches off the light, I can at last feel I have some privacy.

Examples Related to Social Space

Narratives categorized to illustrate social space often contained
references to having one's own room at the hospital or nursing home
and also having given the room a personal character by means of
photos, small pieces of furniture, and other personal belongings. One
nurse at a nursing home said that when patients take their own

belongings to their room, it gave her a feeling that she could not just walk straight into the room—the social space of the patient. The room gave an identity to the patient. Another nurse spoke of the importance of knocking at the patient's door before entering. She said she had to serve as a model for the rest of the staff. This is similar to Barron's (1990) example of how nurses often fail to knock on the bathroom door before entering to help the patient.

In nursing care, it is important to create a social space for patients. For nurses at a nursing home, this is especially necessary for demented patients who cannot protect their own space. The following narrative, related by a nurse at a nursing home, illustrates this.

Example 1

> There was an old demented lady. She usually could not find her way to her room in the ward. We asked her relatives to buy two old-fashioned armchairs. Now we can say to her that the room with the two armchairs is her room—and then she finds her room.

King (1981) states that an individual may try to occupy and own space. In this case the nurse managed to mark the patient's room by using the two old-fashioned armchairs so that the demented patient could distinguish her room (her space) from other rooms. Bakker and Bakker-Rabdau (1973) describe marking of an area to indicate ownership as one type of space-related behavior. It is also possible to interpret the situation from the concept of transaction. The nurse might have realized intuitively that the old demented woman's goal was to find her way to her room—her own space.

One nurse stressed the need for patients to stay in a familiar room, especially when the patient was dying. She said that if her patients did not have a single room, and one patient was going to die, she did not move the dying patient to a single room. Instead, she moved the other patients. She noticed that if she moved the dying patient, he or she would become more confused and look bewildered. The nurse considered it a human right not to be moved to a new place during one's last hours. King (1981) says that alterations, such as a transfer to another room, are a change in social space that may influence the patient's identity and security. Certainly, the nurses' experiences confirm this.

Some nurses observed that demented patients did not always willingly leave their rooms if a new patient arrived. This can be seen, according to Bakker and Bakker-Rabdau (1973) and King (1981), as a sign of indicating ownership of a space. When a patient is admitted to a hospital, the most significant space for the patient is the bed and the bedside table. King (1981) writes that admission to a hospital can lead to a need for the patient to mark off personal territory. The following example illustrates how marked territory can be easily threatened.

Example 2

> I was to hand over the telephone to a patient, and for this I had to take out the plug from the wall. After that, I opened without thinking, one of the drawers in the patient's bedside table in order to put the plug in it. At the same moment, as I opened the drawer, the patient reacted with a deprecating gesture. I happened to glance into the drawer. In the drawer, there were two bars of chocolate. The patient had diabetes and took insulin for his high blood sugar level. I felt as if I had looked into someone's keyhole without permission.

Allekian (1973) proposes that this type of intrusion can give the patient a feeling of depersonalization. The related situation is in accordance with King's (1981) experience that hospital personnel often violate the space of the patient.

Social space can have more invisible limits. King (1981) also stresses that space is situational. She writes, "A person's fears, anxieties, joys and pleasure influence the need for space in situations" (p. 37). The following situation, related by a nurse in an anesthetic ward, illustrates this.

Example 3

> An old lady suffered from arterial thrombosis. Therefore, she was to be operated upon, and it was to be performed under local anesthesia. She was quiet and answered me by nodding. However, she told me that she was worried, because she had no feeling in her leg. The operation was successful, and she told me after the operation, that she had a pricking sensation in her leg. For the first time she smiled. We moved her into her bed and began to

take her to the ward. Suddenly she took her blanket and covered
her face. Why? I looked up, and there was the entire operating
staff. They were talking and laughing. I knew they used to hang
around there after the operations. I wondered how the old lady
felt. Was she afraid of losing control or was the staff too pushy
when they stood there and laughed?

The nurse who told the story explained that the old lady did not
notice the staff before the operation because, at that time, she was
too worried about the operation and her leg. Possibly, her space was
limited due to the stressful situation. She also acted to protect her
limited space from the trespassers—the laughing staff. The situation
shows how staff can violate the patient's space psychologically and
unintentionally. This space-related situation is similar in content to
Minckley's (1968) observations of 600 patients in a recovery room.
Some of the patients pulled covers over their faces, perhaps to get
away from intrusion of their space. Minckley also reported that some
patients showed anger when the staff were joking and laughing.

Allekian (1973) suggests that intrusion into social space can be
more anxiety provoking for patients than intrusion into personal
space. People who enter a hospital may be mentally prepared for
intrusion into intimate space and personal space—for example, in
situations in which they may have to be helped with personal hygiene. However, the effects of intrusions of a more invisible character
against social space, such as having to sleep in a room with people
one does not know and not being able to have some privacy, may not
be so easily tolerated. People may not be as well prepared for this type
of intrusion.

The Concept of Space and
Its Implication for Nursing

The narratives address the interpretation of different signs and
reactions from patients regarding their experience of space. It is
obvious that the person's perception of space is related to the situation and the interaction between the actors. In institutions such as
hospitals and nursing homes, there are many situations and phenomena that can lead to patients' experiencing both threat to their space

and the actual loss of space. If the space of the patient is maintained, the patient might feel more safe and secure.

The narratives both demonstrate the importance of nurses' choosing appropriate strategies for space management and control and provide specific implications for nursing practice. The following statements identify strategies that can be implemented to respect and increase a patient's perception of space:

1. Helping the patient with washing, dressing, and other personal care without threatening the intimate space
2. Helping the elderly patient to show positive feelings of love without experiencing it as a threat to intimate and personal space
3. Helping the patient mark personal and social space
4. Being aware that the patient's space should not be threatened unnecessarily

Discussion

The narratives come from nursing practice and illustrate, in a concrete way, the content of the concept of space. In this way, practice enriches understanding of the theoretical concept, and the theoretical concept enriches practice. Nurses can use the concept to describe and interpret what they see and do when practicing their profession, and that way disseminate knowledge of the concept of space from King's framework. It is also evident from the narratives that concepts in the framework are related. Clearly, this is the case with transaction.

In addition, the narratives demonstrate ways to achieve contextual understanding of King's (1981) definition of space and the importance of space for nursing care. In her definition of space, King states that individuals try to occupy space. The different examples illuminate this statement at several levels. In addition, the concept of perception, which is of major significance in King's framework, is also stressed in the definition of space. In the situations related here, perception is a main variable because the patient's interpretation of space is often connected to how she or he perceived the situation in question.

In Bakker and Bakker-Rabdau's (1973) definition of space, there are four main words: *expert, control, responsibility,* and *initiative.*

These words can be connected to the situations related earlier. Many of them showed that patients had no responsibility for their own person and for the circumstances around them, had no control over the situation, could not take any initiative, or were not regarded as experts. Nurses should be aware of these circumstances and implement strategies to increase the patient's ability to be an expert, take initiative and be responsible, and gain control over the situation.

Bakker and Bakker-Rabdau's (1973) perspective of space is a good fit with King's (1981) philosophical assumptions about human beings and expands King's description of space. According to King, space is personal and unique for every person. This means that if space is unique for every person, it is the person who is the expert in defining the need for space. King also states that "space is subjective and identifies what is *mine*" (p. 137). Marking off what is "mine" is a way to control the situation and have responsibility for one's own space. Furthermore, King identifies that nurses should assess the patient's perception of space, which involves and respects initiatives that the patient takes for privacy.

Relationship of Theory and Practice

The question remains how the concept of space can be connected to King's (1981) theory of goal attainment and used to improve the quality of nursing practice. The essence of King's theory is that nurses interact purposefully and mutually with the patients to establish goals and explore and agree on means to achieve goals. Data from this study suggest that the nurse has to interact with the patient to assess how the patient perceives threats against intimate, personal, and social space. The nurse and the patient have to share thoughts and feelings and mutually move toward a positive experience of space, which will improve the patient's health outcome.

Evaluation

Whall (1989) states that studies that examine concepts of nursing's conceptual models are important. Silva and Sorrell (1992) formulated several evaluation criteria to verify nursing theories that can be used for evaluation of concepts in a nursing conceptual model.

Silva and Sorrell stated that personal experiences of a particular phenomenon can be used to validate derived hypotheses. The narratives related by nurses generated statements about strategies needed for understanding the concepts of space in relation to nursing care. In this type of study, the validity is, according to Sandelowski (1986), subject oriented. This means that it is the informants' experience of the investigated phenomena that is important. The credibility in the study was demonstrated when the nurses spontaneously recognized each other's narratives as examples of the concept of space and agreed on its implications for nursing care. According to Silva and Sorrell (1992), sharing examples, as the nurses did in the study, is a way to confirm the validity of a concept. From that point of view, the examples give validity to the concept of space in King's (1981) framework and its implication for nursing care.

Philosophical Implications

Within philosophy there are three existing criteria of truth—correspondence, coherence, and pragmatic truth. The correspondence criterion of truth refers to statements that correspond to the objective world, whereas the coherence criterion of truth relates to unity, consistency, and internal logic. The pragmatic criterion refers to practical consequences (Kvale, 1989; Silva & Sorrell, 1992). Use of the correspondence criterion has often been practiced within logical empiricism, whereas the criteria of coherence and pragmatism have been emphasized within historicism.

Testing of theory and evaluation of conceptual models raises questions of philosophical assumptions about the validity of truth. Up to now, most of the testing of theories and evaluation of conceptual models of nursing has been related to the criterion of correspondence in the sphere of logical empiricism (Silva & Sorrell, 1992). There is a need for developing methods for validation through the criteria of coherence and pragmatism. According to Sandelowski (1991), the use of narratives stresses validity, which refers to the criterion of coherence, mostly because of its lifelike character. The study presented attempts to address epistemological and methodological questions of validity with regard to coherence and pragmatism.

Theory-Building Implications

According to Walker and Avant (1988), there exist three approaches to theory building—analysis, synthesis, and derivation—which can also be relevant for refining and evaluating concepts in a nursing conceptual model. Analysis is especially useful where there is existing theoretical literature (Walker & Avant, 1988). In the area of the concept of space, there exists a great deal of literature. This study can be seen as an example of analyzing a concept in King's (1981) systems framework in relation to the nursing discipline. Walker and Avant (1988, see Table 2.1, p. 26) state that the purpose of the analysis is to "clarify the use, nature, and properties of the concept." The related narratives highlight the use and nature of the concept of space: For example, the nurse must develop strategies for helping the patient with personal care, strategies for helping the elderly patient to show positive feelings of love, and strategies for helping the patient mark off personal and social space; the nurse must also develop an increased awareness so that a patient's space is not threatened unnecessarily. In that way, the concept of space has been extended as King (1981) has outlined it in her systems framework.

Chenitz and Swanson (1984) state that many nursing conceptual models rely on concepts borrowed from other disciplines. They emphasize the need for integrating these "borrowed" concepts into nursing; otherwise, it is not the nursing discipline that will emerge but more the discipline from which the borrowed concepts originate. Fawcett (1989) points out the need to ensure logical congruence when the borrowed concepts are linked with nursing conceptual models. One advantage of King's (1981) framework is that King has begun the laborious work of integrating some important concepts into the nursing discipline. King's framework can, therefore, be seen as a guide to integrate different concepts into the discipline.

Future Directions

The study gives implications for verifying the concept of space through direct application to nursing practice. Understanding of concepts is demonstrated by the ability to apply knowledge in new situations. Several strategies were suggested to connect knowledge of space to nursing practice. Conducting research that examines the relationship between perception of space and space intervention on health outcome is a logical next step. It would also be possible to deduce theories related to space from King's (1981) framework, and King supports the derivation of other theories from the systems framework. Finally, the method of critical incidents, told in a narrative way, offers possibilities of validating truth in the philosophical sphere of coherence and pragmatism. Investigation and evaluation of other concepts in King's framework, using this method and others, will greatly enhance the scientific basis of the discipline. Nursing is challenged to continue in these directions.

References

Acton, G., Irvin, B., & Hopkins, B. (1991). Theory-testing research: Building the science. *Advances in Nursing Science, 14*(1), 52-61.

Allekian, C. (1973). Intrusions of territory and personal space. *Nursing Research, 22*(3), 236-241.

Altman, I. (1975). *The environment and social behavior: Privacy, personal space, territory, crowding.* Monterey, CA: Brooks/Cole.

Bakker, C., & Bakker-Rabdau, M. (1973). *No trespassing! Explorations in human territoriality.* San Francisco: Chandler & Sharp.

Barron, A. (1990). The right to personal space. *Nursing Times, 86*(27), 28-32.

Benner, P. (1984). *From novice to expert: Excellence and power in clinical nursing practice.* Menlo Park, CA: Addison-Wesley.

Chenitz, C., & Swanson, J. (1984). Surfacing nursing process: A method for generating nursing theory from practice. *Journal of Advanced Nursing, 9*(2), 205-215.

Fawcett, J. (1989). *Analysis and evaluation of conceptual models of nursing* (2nd ed.). Philadelphia: F. A. Davis.

Flanagan, J. (1949). Critical requirements: A new approach to employee evaluation. *Personnel Psychology, 2*(4), 419-425.

Flanagan, J. (1954). The critical incident technique. *Psychological Bulletin, 51*(4), 327-358.

Gonot, P. (1989). Imogene M. King's conceptual framework of nursing. In J. Fitzpatrick & A. Whall (Eds.), *Conceptual models of nursing: Analysis and application* (2nd ed., pp. 271-283). Norwalk, CT: Appleton & Lange.

Greenwood, E. (1957). Attributes of a profession. *Social Work, 2*(3), 45-55.

Hall, E. (1966). *The hidden dimension: Man's use of space in public and private.* London: The Bodley Head.

Hollmerus-Nilsson, I. (1985). *Safety and space: A semantic and theoretical analysis of the concepts of safety and space and the principle of safety and its implication for nursing* (Research Report 7). Helsingfor, Finland: Helsingfor Swedish Nursing Institute.

King, I. (1981). *A theory for nursing: Systems, concepts, process.* New York: John Wiley.

King, I. (1986). *Curriculum and instruction in nursing: Concepts and process.* Norwalk, CT: Appleton-Century-Crofts.

Kvale, S. (1989). To validate is to question. In S. Kvale (Ed.), *Issues of validity in qualitative research* (pp. 73-92). Lund, Sweden: Studentlitteratur.

Minckley, B. (1968). Space and place in patient care. *American Journal of Nursing, 68*(3), 510-516.

Rooke, L. (1990). *Nursing and theoretical structures of nursing. A didactic attempt to develop the practice of nursing.* Published doctoral thesis, University of Lund, Department of Educational Research, Lund, Stockholm, Sweden: Almquist & Wiksell Int.

Sandelowski, M. (1986). The problem of rigor in qualitative research. *Advances in Nursing Science, 8*(3), 27-37.

Sandelowski, M. (1991). Telling stories: Narrative approaches in qualitative research. *Image: Journal of Nursing Scholarship, 23*(3), 161-166.

Silva, M. C. (1986). Research testing nursing theory: State of the art. *Advances in Nursing Science, 9*(1), 1-11.

Silva, M. C., & Rothart, D. (1984). An analysis of changing trends in philosophies of science on nursing theory development and testing. *Advances in Nursing Science, 6*(2), 1-13.

Silva, M. C., & Sorrell, J. M. (1992). Testing of nursing theory: Critique and philosophical expansion. *Advances in Nursing Science, 14*(4), 12-23.

Walker, L., & Avant, K. (1988). *Strategies for theory constructing in nursing* (2nd ed.). Norwalk, CT: Appleton & Lange.

Whall, A. (1989). Nursing science: The process and the products. In J. Fitzpatrick & A. Whall (Eds.), *Conceptual models of nursing: Analysis and application* (2nd ed., pp. 1-14). Norwalk, CT: Appleton & Lange.

8

Family Health
as Derived From
King's Framework

MONA NEWSOME WICKS

King (1983) advocates using her open systems framework and theory of goal attainment to explore families and family health and views health and family as major concepts in the framework. Furthermore, nursing research and practice literature support using the framework to study and care for families (Frey, 1989; Gonot, 1986; Wicks, 1992). The purpose of this chapter is to present a family health theory derived from King's conceptual framework. Discussion describing theory development and preliminary data from test of the theory is included. Although the theory was developed to study families coping with chronic lung disease, it may have broader utility with regard to understanding family health.

Family Health as
the Goal of Nursing

Health is the major focus of King's (1981) conceptual framework. The goal of nursing is to assist clients during times of crisis, through assessment and mutual goal setting to facilitate adjustment to stressors (King, 1983). Thus the goal of family nursing is family health, where health is defined as "a dynamic life experience of a human being, which implies continuous adjustment to stressors in the internal and external environment through optimum use of one's resources to achieve maximum potential for daily living" (King, 1981, p. 5). Families, like individuals, require health (adjustment to internal and external stressors) for successful interpersonal and social role functioning (King, 1981, pp. 3, 4). In addition, family health is culture specific in that the social functions of families are embedded in the cultural norms and values of each group (King, 1981, 1983). King clearly defines individual health. However, within her conceptual framework, individuals are defined as interacting personal systems that form interpersonal and social systems. Consequently, just as individuals experience health, so do groups of individuals, such as families. The nursing care of interpersonal and social systems is well supported in King's writings. By defining family health in terms of functioning, King's definition parallels behavioral theories of family health.

Understanding family health within King's (1981) framework also requires examining her definition of family. King characterizes families as both interpersonal and social systems. Family is broadly defined as a small group of individuals bound together by a common purpose who help in the socialization of children (King, 1983, p. 179). Thus families as transmitters of norms and values are social systems. However, families are categorized as interpersonal systems when group interactions are the focus (King, 1983, p. 180). Within the theory of goal attainment, family as an interpersonal system is "client" in the nurse-client interaction (King, 1983, p. 180). Exploring family health in chronic illness involves examining interacting individuals coping with a lifelong stressor. Consequently, investigating family health in chronic illness involves interpersonal system analyses. However, within systems theory, each system influences the others because interaction occurs across the fluid boundaries of all systems. Hence personal systems (individuals) influence and are influenced by interpersonal systems (dyads and triads, such as families) and social systems (e.g., religious institutions, work organizations, political systems, educational systems, etc.). Like most family systems approaches, this theory has three generic features: a unitary conceptualization of families, the existence of an optimal functioning state (optimal family health), and discussion regarding the openness of the family system (Whall, 1991, p. 320). Examining family systems or the family unit is consistent with King's work because of her inclusion of interpersonal systems (dyads, triads, etc.) within the framework. Within King's (1981, 1983) framework and theory, the client includes patients *and* families. Conceptual congruence between this middle-range theory of family health and King's open systems framework requires the inclusion of both patients (personal systems) and families (interpersonal systems) as appropriate units of analyses because of the influence of the whole on the parts and vice versa.

Chronic caregiving may serve as an individual (personal) and family (interpersonal) systems stressor. Caregiving may have positive as well as negative family system effects (Raveis, Siegel, & Sudit, 1989). Not only is there the potential to strain or strengthen marital relationships and relationships with children, interactions with extended family may also be affected. Research suggests that patients with chronic obstructive pulmonary disease (COPD) and their caregivers interact less with adult children and grandchildren because of illness-related physical limitations and emotional responses (Wicks, 1992). Intergenerational care may, in fact, be multigenerational. Some caregiving families simultaneously cope with child rearing and parent care, whereas others cope with frail parents or in-laws, a chronically ill or frail child, and their own chronic illness. Caring for one chronically ill member potentially alters family dynamics across all generations because families tend to be open systems. For example, inadequate parental coping may negatively influence children socialized in chronic care families, especially when there are multiple competing individual or family stressors. Likewise, a positive caregiving experience, in the context of adequate coping and resources, might positively influence parental socialization of and interactions with children. Chronic illness may potentially hinder or strengthen sibling bonds and impede an ill child's emotional and physical growth and development as well as the development of the family as a whole (Thibodeau, 1988). Disrupted family patterns, conflict, and compromised family health may result when parental expectations for a chronically ill child and their well sibling(s) differ. Thus it seems likely that caregiving experiences do influence the entire family system.

Coping may influence family health (King, personal communication, November 18, 1989). For example, children experiencing stress within caregiving families (in the context of inadequate coping) might manifest altered school performance, and adults might experience impaired job performance or a strained relationship. Families undergoing crisis struggle to achieve a balance and fit at both the individual-to-family and family-to-community levels of functioning (McCubbin & McCubbin, 1987b). Consequently, chronic illness potentially influences health at the personal, interpersonal, and social systems levels.

Perceptions, time, stress, and stressors are among the concepts included in King's framework that have been included in caregiving research. King (1983) proposes that too many stressors may create family crisis, resulting in the need for professional intervention (p. 182). Family caregivers often juggle multiple competing roles— for example, spouse, parent, employee, and so on (Chiriboga, Weiler, & Nielsen, 1989). Like King, family theorists predict that "in crisis situations, the pile up of stressors and strains is related to family adaptation [health]" (McCubbin & McCubbin, 1987a, p. 17).

Extension of King's broad formulations regarding families and family health resulted in theory development and subsequent testing. Operationally defining variables in a manner consistent with King's framework concepts provides an indirect test of the conceptual framework (Fawcett, 1989). King (1983) defines family health in relation to adequate social role functioning. Thus examining family functioning as a measure of family health is congruent with King's formulations.

Concept Relationships

A theory of family health was developed using King's conceptual framework, existing research, and the author's clinical experience with chronic care families. Key concepts included in the theory are perception, time, stress, and stressors. Although King (personal communication, November 18, 1989) believes that coping may influence family health, the concept of coping was omitted from initial tests of the theory to improve subject participation and decrease the number of instruments included in the study. Sexton (1983) has suggested limiting study variables to enhance study participation among chronically ill patients and their families.

Figures 8.1 depicts relationships between concepts (derived from King's conceptual framework) and variables measured in a test of the theory. The concepts perception, time, stress, stressors, and family health (Figure 8.1A) become perception of symptom severity, time since diagnosis, caregiver burden, concurrent family stressors, and family functioning, respectively, in Figure 8.1 Model C. Within the proposed theory, perception of symptom severity is related to caregiver stress (burden), and time is related to both caregiver stress and perceptions of symptom severity. In addition, stress is influenced by the number of family stressors. Figure 8.1 Model A illustrates where coping fits into the theory. Coping, particularly family emotional and material resources, may influence how perception of symptom severity, time since diagnosis, caregiver stress, and family stressors affect family health. Figure 8.1 Model B represents the model as it was empirically tested, without the concept of coping. Perception and time are personal system concepts, whereas stress and stressors (discussed within the concept of stress) are from the interpersonal system. Suggestions of relationships between time, stress, stressors, perception, and family health are implicit and explicit throughout King's formulations. However, because of the level of abstraction inherent in conceptual frameworks, neither the magnitude nor the direction of concept relationships is addressed (Fawcett, 1989).

Stress is necessary for families to function in society (King, 1983). The statement that an individual's response to stress is influenced by stressors, the time of the event, and the perceptions of the event

Conceptual Model A

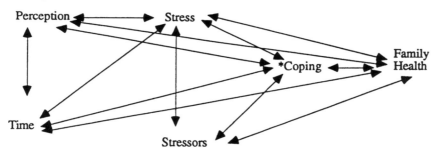

Conceptual Model B

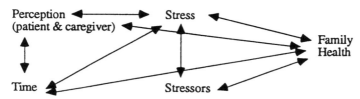

Study Variables C

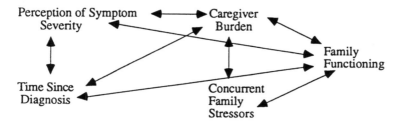

Figure 8.1. Models of Relationships Between Concepts and Variables Included in the
Study of Family Health in Families of Patients With Chronic Obstructive
Pulmonary Disease

NOTE: Arrows represent relationships, not causation.
*Coping was added to the model at the suggestion of Imogene King. Coping is omitted
from models B and C.

supports relationships proposed within the family health theory
(King, 1981, p. 98). Additional support for the contribution of stress

and stressors to family health is implied in King's (1981, 1983) reference to health as a process of adjusting to stressors, and therefore stress, through maximal use of resources to function in one's social roles. Thus family health as family functioning is consistent with King's theoretical perspective (Frey, 1989). Furthermore, King (1983) believes that an individual's perception of what others are perceiving (i.e., family perceptions) about the state of their health may influence and reflect the individual members' perceptions (p. 181). Because the family is the immediate environment of the ill person, family perceptions of an individual's illness must be assessed (King, 1981). King (1983) asserts that time influences perceptions about present events (perception of symptom severity) and may influence a family's behavior (adjustment to the chronic illness as a stressor, which produces stress and influences family health).

When there are disturbances in the normative patterns of interactions, family functioning is disrupted, and professional intervention may be needed (King, 1981, p. 83). A theoretical model that explores relationships between perception of symptom severity, time since diagnosis, caregiver stress, family stressors, and family health or functioning (Figure 8.1C) is consistent with King's framework and family theory and is supported by extant family care research (as will be demonstrated in the next section). King's conceptual framework was used to select instruments and predict relationships as well as to construct a family health theory. Therefore, the validity of King's conceptual framework was tested.

Examining family health provides data about how families respond to life changes and catastrophes (Bishop, Epstein, Keitner, Miller, & Srinivasan, 1986; McCubbin & McCubbin, 1987b). Families may perceive chronic illnesses, such as COPD, as catastrophic, leading to financial strain, altered marital relations, and social isolation. The lifestyle changes experienced by COPD patients and their caregivers have been documented (Sexton & Munro, 1985, 1988; Wicks, 1987). However, the impact of COPD on family systems has not been adequately addressed. For COPD families, social isolation and the need for emotional reserve (to control symptoms) may result in altered family dynamics beyond the caregiver-care recipient dyad.

The relevance of King's conceptual framework for COPD care-giving families is clear. COPD is a progressive disorder with symptoms worsening over *time*. In addition, *perceptions* about symptoms may contribute to individual *stress*. Progressive dependence, frequent infections, and social withdrawal potentially alter family dynamics, including roles, behavior, and communication. Thus patient and caregiver perceptions of the symptoms may influence *family health*. COPD takes place in the context of day-to-day family activities, including developmental and situational *stressors*, that may influence the family's response to the illness.

Empirical Support
for Model Concepts

Evidence suggests that chronic illnesses, such as COPD, disrupt normal family patterns (McCubbin & McCubbin, 1987b; Pless & Satterwhite, 1973; Roberts & Feetham, 1982). Studies supporting the relationships between family health and perception of symptom severity and time have been published. Among caregiving families of cystic fibrosis patients, higher functioning scores were found in families who correctly predicted illness severity (Venters, 1981). Families caring for a member with severe traumatic brain injuries reported greater decreases in functioning over 2 years than did families whose member had less severe injuries (Evans, Bishop, & Ousley, 1992). In addition, families of dialysis, myelodysplasia, and spinal cord injury patients reported decreasing health over time (Kaye, Bray, Gracely, & Levinson, 1989; McGowan & Roth, 1987; Roberts & Feetham, 1982). Although concurrent stressors unrelated to caregiving (day-to-day hassles and strains such as financial and marital strain, etc.) have been found to create the greatest stress for caregivers, the relationship between family functioning and concurrent stressors has not been studied (Chiriboga et al., 1989).

No studies have been published that have specifically examined the theoretical relationships depicted in Figure 8.1C. Consequently, the study model was tested using a correlational-multiple regression design. Data partially supported the family health theory derived from King's (1981) framework. In a test of the family health model, COPD families ($N = 140$) were interviewed and completed a self-report family functioning instrument. The instrument, the Family Assessment Device (Epstein, Baldwin, & Bishop, 1981), measures several aspects of family functioning, including family roles, communication, and general functioning. A major assumption of the study was that COPD family health or functioning would be influenced by the illness. Among COPD families, mean functioning scores were less than optimal (at the cutoff of healthy and unhealthy). However, more than 40% of sample family scores were not healthy when compared with previously established healthy functioning scores. Family scores could not be attributed to COPD as a stressor because no pre-illness family health scores were available. However, interview data revealed that the majority of patients and caregivers directly attributed multiple negative family outcomes (such as social isolation and financial strain) to the illness (Wicks, 1992). In addition, study variables explained 28% of the variance in family health scores ($p < .05$), although the contribution of time to the family health model was not statistically significant.

Relationships between family health and perception of symptom severity, time since diagnosis, caregiver stress, and concurrent family stressors were also tested. COPD family health was related to perception of symptom severity. Most patient-reported symptoms and several caregiver-reported symptoms were related to family health. Less healthy families had caregivers and patients who perceived more frequent patient symptoms, with correlations ranging from $r = .18$ to $r = .34$, $p < .05$. Family health was not significantly related to time, as predicted in the family health theory. Time was significantly related neither to perceived symptom severity nor to caregiver stress. However, less healthy families had more burdened caregivers ($r = .32$, $p < .05$) and more stressors as predicted ($r = .30$, $p < .05$). In addition, as hypothesized, patients with more frequent patient-reported and caregiver-reported symptoms had more burdened caregivers (correlations ranging from .24-.65, $p < .05$). Thus family health was influenced by perception, stress, and stressors as predicted within the family health theory derived from King's conceptual framework.

Conclusion

Conceptual frameworks provide direction for organizing thoughts and data and for formulating questions and interpreting data (Fawcett, 1989). King's theoretical formulations guided concept development, operational definitions, and instrument selection. Although relationships between framework variables are suggested, King does not delineate their direction or magnitude. The broad nature of conceptual frameworks requires that the magnitude and direction of concept relationship be defined by systematic investigation (Fawcett, 1989). Consequently, a middle-range theory of family health was proposed and tested. As predicted, family health was influenced by multiple individual as well as family factors. Family health was influenced by perception, stress, and stressors but not by time. Further testing of the theory is needed to explore its usefulness with families adjusting to other chronic illnesses. Family theorists advocate the use of a "health care oriented family systems" perspective to explore family health in chronic illness (McCubbin & McCubbin, 1987b). King's framework, from which the theory of family health was derived, fits this criterion. In addition, this family health theory supports the usefulness of developing middle-range theories from existing nursing frameworks.

References

Bishop, D. S., Epstein, N. B., Keitner, G. I., Miller, I. W., & Srinivasan, S. V. (1986). Stroke: Morale, family functioning, health status, and functional capacity. *Archives of Physical Medicine & Rehabilitation, 67*(2), 84-87.

Chiriboga, D. A., Weiler, P. G., & Nielsen, K. (1989). The stress of caregivers. *Journal of Applied Social Sciences, 13*(1), 119-141.

Epstein, N. B., Baldwin, L. M., & Bishop, D. S. (1981). McMaster model of family functioning: A review of the normal family. In F. Walsh (Ed.), *Normal family process* (pp. 115-141). New York: Guilford.

Evans, R. L., Bishop, D. S., & Ousley, R. T. (1992). Providing care to persons with physical disability: Effect on family caregivers. *American Journal of Physical Medicine & Rehabilitation, 71*(3), 140-144.

Fawcett, J. (1989). *Analysis and evaluation of conceptual models of nursing.* Philadelphia: F. A. Davis.

Frey, M. A. (1989). Social support and health: A theoretical formulation derived from King's conceptual framework. *Nursing Science Quarterly,* 2(3), 138-148.

Gonot, P. W. (1986). Family therapy as derived from King's conceptual model. In A. L. Whall (Ed.), *Family therapy for nursing: Four approaches* (pp. 33-48). Norwalk, CT: Appleton-Century-Crofts.

Kaye, J., Bray, S., Gracely, E. J., & Levinson, S. (1989). Psychological adjustment to illness and family environment in dialysis patients. *Family Systems Medicine,* 7(1), 77-81.

King, I. M. (1981). *A theory for nursing.* New York: John Wiley.

King, I. M. (1983). King's theory of nursing. In I. W. Clements & F. B. Roberts (Eds.), *Family health: A theoretical approach to nursing care* (pp. 178-188). New York: John Wiley.

McCubbin, H. I., & McCubbin, M. A. (1987a). Family stress theory and assessment: The T-double ABCX model of family adjustment and adaptation. In H. McCubbin & A. Thompson (Eds.), *Family assessment inventories for research and practice* (pp. 3-32). Madison: University of Wisconsin Press.

McCubbin, H. I., & McCubbin, M. A. (1987b). Family system assessment in health care. In H. McCubbin & A. Thompson (Eds.), *Family assessment inventories for research and practice* (pp. 53-78). Madison: University of Wisconsin Press.

McGowan, M. B., & Roth, S. (1987). Family functioning and functional independence in spinal cord injury adjustment. *Paraplegia, 25,* 357-365.

Pless, I. B., & Satterwhite, B. (1973). A measure of family functioning and its application. *Social Science and Medicine, 7,* 613-621.

Raveis, V. H., Siegel, K., & Sudit, M. (1989). Psychological impact of caregiving on the care provider: A critical review of extant research. *Journal of Applied Social Sciences, 13*(1), 40-79.

Roberts, C. S., & Feetham, S. L. (1982). Assessing family functioning scores across three areas of relationships. *Nursing Research, 31*(4), 231-235.

Sexton, D. L. (1983). Some methodological issues in chronic illness research. *Nursing Research, 32*(6), 378-380.

Sexton, D. L., & Munro, B. H. (1985). Impact of a husband's chronic illness (COPD) on the spouse's life. *Research in Nursing and Health, 8,* 83-90.

Sexton, D. L., & Munro, B. H. (1988). Living with chronic illness: The experience of women with chronic obstructive pulmonary disease (COPD). *Western Journal of Nursing Research, 10*(1), 26-44.

Thibodeau, S. M. (1988). Sibling response to chronic illness: The role of the clinical nurse specialist. *Issues in Comprehensive Pediatric Nursing, 11*(1), 17-28.

Venters, M. (1981). Familial coping with chronic and severe childhood illness: The case of cystic fibrosis. *Social Science and Medicine, 15,* 289-297.

Whall, A. L. (1991). Family systems theory: Relationship to nursing conceptual models. In A. L. Whall & J. Fawcett (Eds.), *Family theory development in nursing: State of the science and art* (pp. 317-341). Philadelphia: F. A. Davis.

Wicks, M. N. (1987). *Impact of chronic illness on husbands of women with chronic obstructive pulmonary disease.* Unpublished master's thesis, University of Tennessee, Memphis.

Wicks, M. N. (1992). *Family health in chronic illness.* Unpublished doctoral dissertation, Wayne State University, Detroit, MI.

9

Toward a Theory of Families, Children, and Chronic Illness

MAUREEN A. FREY

Development of theoretical perspectives for understanding the complex factors that contribute to child and family health in the face of chronic illness has increased dramatically in the past 10 years. This is due to the change in emphasis from cure to adjustment and maximizing functioning, from acute to long-term management, and from professional to family and individual responsibility for care. Although nursing plays a major role in the health and health care of children with chronic illness and their families, theoretical perspectives for organizing, delivering, and evaluating that care often come from other disciplines. Although knowledge of child development, physiology, and families is important, a nursing framework ensures that the activities involved in care, and the goals of care, reflect the perspective of nursing.

Imogene King's (1981, 1990) systems framework for nursing provides structure and function for understanding the complex interplay of factors that influence family and child health when the child has a chronic illness. Structure includes the conceptual orientation of dynamic interaction between personal, interpersonal, and social systems; identification of concepts that are important for understanding systems and their interactions; and specification of health as the goal of nursing. This last aspect of structure is especially important because it is specific to the discipline of nursing.

King's (1981) framework also provides direction for functions of members of the discipline, both scientists and practitioners. Scientists expand the knowledge base of practice by developing and testing hypotheses related to human interactions and health. Practitioners use, evaluate, and refine nursing knowledge in practice situations.

For the past 10 years, I have developed, tested, and continue to refine a theory of family, children, and chronic illness derived from King's (1981) systems framework. The initial formulation focused on the concepts of interaction and health of the family system and individual child. Relevant indicators and measures, consistent with King's perspective, were identified for children with insulin-dependent diabetes mellitus (IDDM) on the basis of review of theoretical, empirical, and clinical literature. The formulation was tested with 107 youths with IDDM between the ages of 10 and 16. Results of that study were used to expand the theory and improve the measurement of child health (Frey, 1988). The most significant addition was inclusion of the behavioral variables general health and illness actions, which were also hypothesized to affect child health.

The revised theory was subsequently tested with 37 youths with IDDM (Frey, 1989). Given the small sample size, statistical testing of the entire theory was not possible. However, correlational analysis indicated that the behavioral concepts were important. Youths with higher levels of general health behavior reported poorer physical and mental status, better functional health, and higher perception of their health than did those with lower levels of general health behavior. In addition, Youths with higher levels of illness management behavior reported better physical and mental status and better metabolic control (an illness indicator) than did those who reported lower levels (Frey, 1993a).

Again, the data were used to revise the theory in terms of indicators and measures, primarily family and child health (Frey, 1993b).

For example, coping, resources, and stressors were added as components of family health. The concept of coping has recently been included in King's (1992) framework. Coping with stressors and using resources are processes related to health (King, 1981). Several additional child health indicators that expanded personal, social, and physical functioning were also included.

Funding was obtained from the Public Health Service, National Institutes of Health, National Center for Nursing Research (R29NR02243) to test the revised theory with two groups of children, those with IDDM and asthma, over a 5-year period. This provided a comparison group as well as the opportunity to look at change over time via longitudinal design. In this chapter, the first wave of data is presented for both illness groups to determine if illness factors (duration, age at onset, illness status, child's perception of severity), social support (parents' general support, support regarding the illness, and satisfaction with support; child's general support, support regarding the illness, satisfaction with support), family health (adaptability, cohesion, resources, coping, stressors), and health actions (child's general health and illness management behaviors) explain a significant amount of the variance in child health outcome (role competence, school attendance, school performance, perception of health, physical and mental status) as predicted by the theory (see Figure 9.1).

Methods

Sample

The convenience sample was drawn from the registries of the pediatric diabetes and pulmonary clinics of a large teaching hospital. Inclusion criteria were children (a) between the ages of 10 and 16 years, (b) diagnosed for more than 6 months, and (c) with no other significant health or developmental problems. Youths in the IDDM group were specifically asked about history of asthma or any other respiratory pathology. Youths were not excluded if they reported having allergies. For children from two-parent families, both parents were asked to participate. Characteristics of the sample are shown in Table 9.1. Overall, the IDDM and asthma groups are very similar;

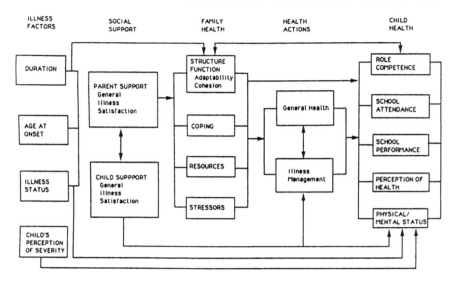

Figure 9.1. Proposed Theory of Families, Children, and Chronic Illness

both are deemed representative of the children who receive specialized health care at the medical center.

Instruments

Data were collected by a number of established, self-report scales consistent with the indicators of concepts in the theory. Parents completed FACES III (Olson, Portner, & Lavee, 1985), Coping Health Inventory for Children (CHIP) (McCubbin, McCubbin, & Cauble, 1987), Family Inventory of Life Events and Changes (FILE) (McCubbin & Patterson, 1987), Family Inventory of Resources for Management (FIRM) (McCubbin & Comeau, 1987), and the Norbeck Social Support Questionnaire (Norbeck, 1984; Norbeck, Lindsey, & Carrieri, 1981, 1983). Children completed FACES III, Denyes Self-Care Practice Instrument (DSCPI) (Denyes, 1980), Diabetes (or Asthma) Self-Care Practice Instrument (Fitzpatrick, 1991), Denyes Health Status Instrument (DHSI) (Denyes, 1980), Self-Perception Profile for Children (SPPC) (Harter, 1985), and the Brief Symptom Inventory (BSI) (Derogatis & Spencer, 1982). Additional information was obtained during family interviews and from medical records.

TABLE 9.1   Characteristics of the Sample

Characteristics	IDDM[a]		Asthma[b]	
	M	SD	M	SD
Children				
Age (years)	12.6	1.5	12.9	1.8
Age at diagnosis (years)	7.9	3.7	4.2	2.8
Length of illness (years)	4.6	3.2	8.7	3.3
Families				
Hollingshead score	45.4	12.3	48.7	12.4
Two parent	76%		69%	
Income > $25,000/year	85%		86%	
Ethnic affiliation				
African American	4%		10%	
European American	92%		90%	
Other	4%		0%	

a. Females: $n = 22$; males: $n = 28$; mothers: $n = 49$; fathers: $n = 38$.
b. Females: $n = 11$; males: $n = 28$; mothers: $n = 39$; fathers: $n = 27$.

Procedures

Data were collected during in-home interviews by trained research assistants. Descriptive statistics, t tests, and regression techniques were used to analyze data.

Results

T-test analysis was used to determine if there were differences between the illness groups on the measured variables. Significant differences are shown in Table 9.2. Differences were most notable for youths in the areas of general health and illness behaviors, dimensions of role competence, perception of health, and several illness variables. Family differences occurred in relation to resources and stressors, although the samples were extremely similar on other socioeconomic indicators.

A series of multiple regression analyses using backward elimination were done for each illness group using the child health outcomes as dependent variables. Because of the large number of variables in the model and relatively small sample size, not all variables were

TABLE 9.2   Comparison of Illness Groups

| | IDDM | | Asthma | | |
Variable	M	SD	M	SD	t*
Family					
Resources: mother	111.6	14.5	99.1	14.2	3.93
Resources: father	113.6	14.1	95.8	9.6	5.97
Stressors: family	12.0	5.6	15.0	5.9	2.41
Youths					
Duration of illness (years)	4.6	3.2	8.7	3.3	5.83
Illness support	9.4	1.9	8.3	2.9	2.19
General health behavior	76.9	10.9	66.6	14.6	3.65
Illness management	78.1	12.6	63.4	12.9	5.17
Social acceptance	3.2	0.6	2.8	0.7	3.01
Behavioral competence	3.2	0.6	2.8	0.5	2.99
Self-worth	3.4	0.5	3.0	0.5	2.72
Perception of health	81.6	10.7	74.4	12.1	2.85

$p < .05$.

included in the analysis. Exclusion of variables was based on low weights as indicated by preliminary canonical analysis correlations and theoretical redundancy. Results of the analyses are shown in Tables 9.3 and 9.4 for the IDDM and asthma groups, respectively.

Taken together, family, illness, and health behavior variables, singly and in combination, explained from 13% to 72% of the variance in child health. In general, explained variances tended to be greater for the asthma group, especially in the area of role competence. In addition, there was a different pattern of predictors for the two groups. Predictors of child health for youths with IDDM were general health and illness management behaviors, illness variables of age at diagnosis, and duration of illness and, less frequently, the family health variables of cohesion and adaptability. Mother's general support and child's satisfaction with general support were the only significant social support variables that predicted a dimension of health in the IDDM sample.

In contrast, the family health variables of adaptability, cohesion, coping, resources, and stressors and social support variables were much more likely to be predictors of child health outcome for the asthma group. General health behavior was a significant predictor only of physical and mental status. Neither illness management

TABLE 9.3   Regression Analysis Predicting Health Outcome in Youths With IDDM

Variable	Beta	R^2 [a]	p
Scholastic competence			
General health behavior	.04	.32	< .001
Social competence			
General health behavior	.04	.32	< .001
Illness management	−.02		
Athletic competence			
General health behavior	−.55	.29	.002
Gender[b]	.02		
Physical appearance			
Duration of illness	−.13	.39	.001
Age at diagnosis	−.13		
Gender	−.39		
Family cohesion: child's view	−.04		
Behavioral competence			
Family cohesion: mother's view	.06	.20	.003
Self-worth			
General health behavior	.01	.49	< .001
Gender	−.30		
Family adaptability: mother's view	.03		
Family cohesion: child's view	.04		
School progress			
Duration of illness	−.25	.24	.003
Age at diagnosis	−.24		
Perception of health			
Mother's general support	1.59	.38	< .001
Child's satisfaction with general support	9.55		
Physical and mental status			
Family cohesion: child's view	−.03	.15	.007

a. Cumulative R^2. Significance of change in R^2 was based on F-ratio.
b. 1 = females; 2 = males.

behavior nor indicators of illness were related to any child health outcome for the asthma sample.

Discussion

The results of the study indicate that various dimensions of illness, social support, family health, and child's health behavior are

TABLE 9.4   Regression Analysis Predicting Health Outcome in Youths With
                Asthma

Variable	Beta	R^2 [a]	p
Scholastic competence			
Mother's coping	.01	.68	< .001
Father's coping	−.01		
Mother's resources	.01		
Father's resources	.02		
Family stressors	.03		
Social competence			
Father's resources		.57	< .001
Athletic competence			
Mother's general support	−.07	.71	< .001
Mother's satisfaction with general support	.33		
Father's cohesion	−.04		
Father's resources	.02		
Physical appearance			
Father's satisfaction with general support	.31	.55	.002
Child's satisfaction with general support	−.30		
Father's resources	.02		
Behavioral competence			
Family adaptability: child's view	−.02	.72	< .001
Family cohesion: mother's view	−.04		
Family cohesion: father's view	−.04		
Mother's resources	.02		
Self-worth			
Father's satisfaction with general support	.34	.58	< .001
Family cohesion: mother's view	−.05		
Mother's resources	.02		
School absences			
Family adaptability: mother's view	.54	.23	.02
School progress			
Family cohesion: father's view	.08	.16	.04
Perception of health			
Mother's satisfaction with general support	8.1 [b]	.13	.02
Physical and mental status			
Child's general support	−.04	.37	< .001
General health behavior	−.01		

a. Cumulative R^2. Significance of change in R^2 was based on F-ratio.
b. Based on ANOVA.

related to child health outcome as predicted by the theory. Because
the theory was derived from King's (1981) systems framework, this
provides empirical data in support of the framework. The findings

also provide direction for assessment of and interventions to improve health outcomes in children with IDDM and asthma as well as further theory development.

Previous research has not resulted in a clear picture of health in these populations, perhaps because of the use of illness and metabolic control as measures of health status (Frey, 1993a). From King's perspective, health is multidimensional, with emphasis on functional role and perception. In this study, definition and measurement of functional role took into consideration several aspects of personal and social development, and youths were asked to evaluate their own health status. A general, rather than an illness-specific, measure of physical and mental status was also included so as to move away from exclusive focus on the illness.

A somewhat different picture of health emerged for the two groups. Youths with IDDM reported higher levels of social acceptance, behavioral competence, self-worth (indicators of functional health), and perception of health but no difference in physical and mental status compared to youths with asthma. These findings certainly support the need to move beyond the physical dimension when assessing health in children with chronic illness. They also show that health of children with asthma may be fairly compromised by the illness, something not always recognized by the general public. Examples of the latter include attitudes and beliefs that asthma will be "outgrown" and/or that it has a major psychological component. These findings can be used by health care professionals to ensure that children and families get the support and services they need, especially in school and community settings.

The other major area where there were differences between the groups was in relation to general health and illness management behaviors. Youths with IDDM reported higher levels of both. In considering the nature of illness management for these two diagnostic groups, it was somewhat surprising that the level of care was higher for the more invasive and personal care associated with IDDM (e.g., injections, blood and urine testing). On the other hand, IDDM care is daily and unrelenting, even in the absence of symptoms related to illness. Asthma management might be more likely to vary on the basis of illness status, activity, or environmental change. Investigation into the meaning and problematic aspects of care for families and youths would be very helpful in understanding identified differences.

Although both illness management and general health behavior were lower for the asthma group, Frey (1993a) has reported a significant relationship between illness and general health behavior in youths with IDDM and youths with asthma across several other samples. This suggests that the difference might not be due simply to the overlap between illness management and general health behavior (e.g., exercise and nutrition) for the IDDM group. Because general health and illness management behaviors are related, promotion of general health remains an important area for assessment and intervention. The longitudinal data should provide important information about how health and illness behaviors covary over time.

On the basis of King's (1981) framework, there was no basis to predict how health outcome would be differentially influenced by the variables included in the theory for the two groups. The clinical literature identifies that family, support, and illness management are important in both. Several clear differences emerged. First was the pattern of predictors. For the asthma group, these were dominated by dimensions of the family system. Although illness in a family member can increase the need for resources and be a major stressor, the measures used in this study tapped personal, financial, social, and community resources and a broad range of stressors for families, far beyond illness. In addition, family adaptability and cohesion tap general and somewhat stable characteristics of families. Taken together, these findings support the importance of illness-specific stressors and need to look beyond them to the broader picture of family development, relationships, lifestyle, and resource base. Although illness management is only one variable in the theory, the absence of its relationship with child health is surprising given the emphasis placed on illness management in clinical practice. Clearly, this is an area for ongoing investigation.

In contrast, child health for the IDDM group was primarily influenced by general health and illness management behaviors. This is an important finding and may account for the higher health status reported by youths with IDDM. It is not clear why the family factors were not significant predictors of health for this group. It is very possible that family influences are less direct than tested in this study or related to temporal, illness, or other factors. Additional analysis may provide clarification of these relationships.

The findings raise questions about the contribution of social support to health. This is surprising given the frequency with which the concept of support and its multiple indicators are related to health outcome in the theoretical and clinical literature. Even the inclusion of illness support and satisfaction with support variables has not increased predictive power. There may be several reasons for this. One explanation might be the theoretical perspective of social support as buffer (i.e., stress perspectives) versus social support as a general protective resource of the family or individual. From both clinical and research experiences with these families and children, it is clear that families do not see themselves as "in crisis" at this point past diagnosis, and many do not consider themselves or their children as "unhealthy" because of the medical diagnosis. A second reason might be that most of the theoretical and measurement work with social support has been done with adults and does not generalize to children and adolescents. However, the child's satisfaction with general support was related to several health outcomes. Although not strong, the findings justify retaining the concept in the theory.

Theoretical Expansion

It is likely that expansion of the theory, although complex and integrative, would greatly enhance understanding of child health outcome, especially for youths with IDDM. Reexamination resulted in identification of several gaps. For example, what does the child bring to the situation? Many characteristics of the family have been considered, but what about the child? What are the indirect relationships between concepts related to health? For example, what factors influence illness status? How do family factors influence illness management and general health behaviors? How does illness management influence illness status?

Direction for theory revision is based on further examination of King's framework. King (1988) states that concepts provide the building blocks of conceptual frameworks and theories. She identifies a number of concepts that are important for understanding personal,

interpersonal, and social systems. In developing knowledge specific
to nursing situations, relevant concepts are selected, their characteristics identified, and relationships validated in research. The
concepts of self, growth and development, and stress were selected
for further understanding the nature and behavior of youths as
personal systems.

King (1981) quotes Jersild's definition of self for nursing:

> "The self is a composite of thoughts and feeling which constitute
> a person's awareness of his individual existence, his conception
> of who and what he is. A person's self is the sum total of all he
> can call his. The self includes, among other things, a system of
> ideas, attitudes, values and commitments. The self is a person's
> total subjective environment. It is a distinctive center of experi-
> ence and significance. The self constitutes a person's inner world
> as distinguished from the outer world consisting of all other
> people and things. The self is the individual as known to the in-
> dividual. It is that to which we refer when we say 'I.' " (pp. 27-28)

Knowledge of how people perceive themselves is essential for nurses
to increase self-awareness in others, especially in times of stressful
life experiences. In addition, expression of self is reflected in patterns
of growth and development and human behavior. King (1981) drew
from the well-known theories of Erikson, Freud, Piaget, Gesell, and
Havighurst in examining the concept of growth and development for
nursing. Understanding the process of growth and development,
positive and negative factors that affect growth and development, and
the relationship between growth and development and behavior is
essential for planning health care and teaching. Moreover, knowledge
of growth and development enables nurses to care for persons across
the life span.

King (1981) identified that placement of concepts across systems
was somewhat arbitrary. For example, although the concept of stress
is discussed in relation to the interpersonal system, it is expressed
from the perspective of the individual. King identified that stress is
ubiquitous. It is a personal and subjective response to persons,
objects, and events called *stressors*. Stress is often reflected in patterns of behavior. Assisting persons to decrease, eliminate, or manage

stress is an important component of nursing care because the ability to adjust to stressors relates to health.

Review of the literature in the areas of chronic illness, in general, and IDDM and asthma, specifically, provides additional support and direction for expanding the focus on self, growth and development, and stress. Many variables that have been investigated in youths— for example, locus of control, self-efficacy, and various personality characteristics—would fit under King's definition of self.

Aspects of self that seem important are motivation and adjustment. Interesting work in the area of children's motivation has been reported by Cox, Cowell, Marion, and Miller (1990). Motivation is based on Deci's cognitive evaluation theory, which suggests that the process of choosing behavior is the primary energy source for setting and meeting goals (Deci, 1975; Deci & Ryan, 1985). Adjustment implies feelings of acceptance and value despite limitations, risks, or changes imposed by illness and its management (Felton & Revenson, 1984; Felton, Revenson, & Hinrichsen, 1984). Motivation and adjustment are consistent with King's (1981) framework because adjustment and motivation, as perceptual-cognitive processes, are specifically identified as influences of behavior and health outcome. Both are subjective, describe capabilities, and reflect values and beliefs.

The impact of chronic illness on development of children and adolescents has been addressed extensively. For the most part, attention has been directed toward psychosocial development and responses to diagnosis and treatment. However, adolescence is characterized by the unique phenomenon of puberty, a time of rapid hormonal, physical, and emotional changes. It is known that chronic illness influences puberty and puberty influences chronic illness. Effects include delay of pubertal development, a change in the expression of illness (sometimes improving, sometimes getting worse), the effectiveness of treatment, and compliance with treatment (Balfour-Lynn, 1985; Burns, Green, & Chase, 1986; Hein, 1987; Ibrahim et al., 1983).

Attention to the biological-hormonal-behavioral link during puberty is due to advances in the emerging field of psychoneuroendocrinology. Research has pointed to the link between hormones and aggression (Olweus, 1986) and sexual behavior (Udry, Billy, Morris,

Groff, & Raj, 1985; Udry, Talber, & Morris, 1986). There has been very little investigation of the link between hormones and other behaviors, such as health actions or illness management. This is an exciting area of research and likely to provide a greater understanding of human behavior, behavior that clearly has short- and long-term implications for health.

Although stress and stressors have been extensively discussed and researched in adult populations, the likelihood that children and youths experience stressors and stress has gained considerable attention (Atkins, 1991; Brady & Grey, 1990; Grey & Hayman, 1987; Newcomb, Huba, & Bentler, 1981; Swearingen & Cohen, 1985). Theory and research in this area have addressed stressful life events (e.g., death of a parent, changing schools), laboratory-induced acute stressors, and physical stress (e.g., puberty or illness). More recently, the trend has been to consider the impact of chronic stress on development and behavior. Several investigators (Chase & Jackson, 1981; Coddington, 1984; Mendez, Yeaworth, York, & Goodwin, 1980) have reported that stress increases with age during adolescence. This certainly suggests a link with hormones, because hormones change greatly during this period also. Nottlemann et al. (1987) found that higher levels of androstenedione (a steroid responsive to stress) in males was associated with more aggressive behavior, adjustment problems, irritability, and impulsivity. Although generally investigated in relation to the stressfulness of adolescence, behavioral changes could also reflect chronic illness.

The concepts of stress, growth and development, adjustment, and motivation are important theoretically, clinically relevant, and empirically grounded and likely to provide better understanding of youths as personal systems and how the personal system influences behavior and health. Knowledge of these important factors will contribute to the science of nursing.

References

Atkins, F. D. (1991). Children's perspective of stress and coping: An integrative review. *Issues in Mental Health Nursing, 12,* 171-178.

Balfour-Lynn, L. (1985). Childhood asthma and puberty. *Archives of Diseases in Childhood, 60,* 231-235.

Brady, M., & Grey, M. (1990). Tools for assessing stress in children. *Journal of Pediatric Health Care, 4*(5), 260-261.

Burns, K. L., Green, P., & Chase, H. P. (1986). Psychosocial correlates of glycemic control as a function of age in youth with insulin-dependent diabetes. *Journal of Adolescent Health Care, 7,* 311-319.

Chase, H. P., & Jackson, G. G. (1981). Stress and sugar control in children with insulin-dependent diabetes mellitus. *Journal of Pediatrics, 98*(6), 1011-1013.

Coddington, R. D. (1984). Measuring the stressfulness of a child's environment. In J. H. Humphrey (Ed.), *Stress in childhood* (pp. 97-126). New York: AMS Press.

Cox, C. L., Cowell, J. M., Marion, L. N., & Miller, E. H. (1990). The health self-determinism index for children. *Research in Nursing & Health, 13,* 237-246.

Deci, E. L. (1975). *Intrinsic motivation.* New York: Plenum.

Deci, E. L., & Ryan, R. M. (1985). *Intrinsic motivation and self-determinism in human behavior.* New York: Plenum.

Denyes, M. J. (1980). Development of an instrument to measure self-care agency in adolescents. *Dissertation Abstracts International, 4,* 1716B. (University Microfilms No. 8025672)

Derogatis, L. R., & Spencer, P. M. (1982). *Administration and procedures: BSI manual—I.* Riderwood, MD: Clinical Psychometric Research.

Felton, B. J., & Revenson, R. A. (1984). Coping with chronic illness: A study of illness controllability and the influence of coping strategies on psychological adjustment. *Journal of Consulting and Clinical Psychology, 52,* 343-353.

Felton, B. J., Revenson, R. A., & Hinrichsen, G. A. (1984). Stress and coping in the explanation of psychological adjustment among chronically ill adults. *Social Science and Medicine, 18,* 889-898.

Fitzpatrick, M. (1991). *Development of an instrument to measure health-deviation self-care in school age children and adolescents with asthma.* Unpublished master's thesis, University of Michigan, Ann Arbor.

Frey, M. A. (1988). *Health and social support in families with children with diabetes mellitus* (Doctoral dissertation, Wayne State University, 1987). *Dissertation Abstracts International, 48,* 4A.

Frey, M. A. (1989). Social support and health: A theoretical formulation derived from King's conceptual framework. *Nursing Science Quarterly, 2,* 138-148.

Frey, M. A. (1993a). *Self-care and health in youths with chronic illness: Directions for research*. Unpublished manuscript.

Frey, M. A. (1993b). A theoretical perspective of family and child health derived from King's conceptual framework for nursing. In S. L. Feetham, S. B. Meister, J. M. Bell, & C. L. Gilliss (Eds.), *The nursing of families* (pp. 30-37). Newbury Park, CA: Sage.

Grey, M., & Hayman, L. L. (1987). Assessing stress in children: Research and clinical implications. *Journal of Pediatric Nursing, 2*(5), 316-327.

Harter, S. (1985). *Manual for the self-perception profile for children*. Denver, CO: University of Denver.

Hein, K. (1987). The interface of chronic illness and the hormonal regulation of puberty. *Journal of Adolescent Health Care, 8*, 530-540.

Ibrahim, I. I., Saker, R., Ghaly, I. M., Abdalla, M. I., Shams El-Din, A. A., Osman, M. I., Helmy, F., El-Meliegy, R., Abu-Zekry, M., & Hafez, S. E. (1983). Endocrine profiles in pediatric andrology: II. Insulin-dependent diabetic adolescents. *Archives of Andrology, 11*, 45-51.

King, I. (1981). *A theory for nursing: Systems, concepts, process*. New York: John Wiley.

King, I. (1988). Concepts: Essential elements of theories. *Nursing Science Quarterly, 16*, 22-25.

King, I. (1990). Health as the goal for nursing. *Nursing Science Quarterly, 3*(3), 123-128.

King, I. (1992). King's theory of goal attainment. *Nursing Science Quarterly, 5*(1), 19-26.

McCubbin, H., & Comeau, J. (1987). Family inventory of resources for management (FIRM). In H. McCubbin & A. Thompson (Eds.), *Family assessment for research and practice* (pp. 144-160). Madison: University of Wisconsin Press.

McCubbin, H., McCubbin, M., & Cauble, A. E. (1987). Coping health inventory for parents (CHIP). In H. McCubbin & A. Thompson (Eds.), *Family assessment for research and practice* (pp. 175-193). Madison: University of Wisconsin Press.

McCubbin, M. A., & Patterson, J. M. (1987). FILE family inventory of life events and changes. In H. McCubbin & A. Thompson (Eds.), *Family assessment inventories for research and practice* (pp. 81-96). Madison: University of Wisconsin Press.

Mendez, L. K., Yeaworth, R. C., York, J. A., & Goodwin, T. (1980). Factors influencing adolescents' perceptions of life change events. *Nursing Research, 29*(6), 384-388.

Newcomb, M. D., Huba, G. J., & Bentler, P. M. (1981). A multidimensional assessment of stressful life events among adolescents: Derivation and correlates. *Journal of Health and Social Behavior, 22*, 400-415.

Norbeck, J. S. (1984). The Norbeck social support questionnaire. In K. E. Barnard, P. A. Brandt, B. S. Raff, & P. Carroll (Eds.), *Social support and families of vulnerable infants* (pp. 45-57). New York: March of Dimes Birth Defects Foundation.

Norbeck, J. S., Lindsey, A. M., & Carrieri, V. L. (1981). The development of an instrument to measure social support. *Nursing Research, 30*, 264-269.

Norbeck, J. S., Lindsey, A. M., & Carrieri, V. L. (1983). Further development of the Norbeck Social Support Questionnaire: Normative data and validity testing. *Nursing Research, 32*, 4-9.

Nottelmann, E. D., Susman, E. J., Inoff-Germain, G., Cutler, G. B., Loriaux, D. L., & Chrousos, G. P. (1987). Developmental processes in early adolescence: Relationships between adolescent adjustment problems and chronologic age, pubertal stage, and puberty-related serum hormone levels. *Journal of Pediatrics, 110*, 473-480.

Olson, D. H., Portner, J., & Lavee, Y. (1985). *FACES III*. St. Paul: University of Minnesota Press.

Olweus, D. (1986). Aggression and hormones: Behavioral relationships with testosterone and adrenaline. In D. Olweus, J. Block, & M. Radke-Yarrow (Eds.), *Development of antisocial and prosocial behavior: Research, theories, and issues* (pp. 51-71). Orlando, FL: Academic Press.

Swearingen, E. M., & Cohen, L. H. (1985). Life events and psychological distress: A prospective study of young adolescents. *Developmental Psychology, 21*(6), 1045-1054.

Udry, J. K., Billy, J. G., Morris, N. M., Groff, T. R., & Raj, M. H. (1985). Serum androgenic hormones motivate sexual behavior in boys. *Fertility and Sterility, 43*, 90-94.

Udry, J. R., Talber, L. M., & Morris, N. M. (1986). Biosocial foundations for adolescent female sexuality. *Demography, 23*, 217-230.

10

Using King's Interacting Systems Framework for Research on Parents of Children With Neural Tube Defect

ELIZABETH F. HOBDELL

Psychological preparation during pregnancy involves mothers' and fathers' fantasies of an ideal child. The discrepancy between this ideal and the actual child must be resolved by all parents (Drotar, Baskiewicz, Irvin, Kennell, & Klaus, 1975; Solnit & Stark, 1961). The birth of a child with neural tube defect accentuates this natural loss of the ideal child. Mothers and fathers may not only have seen the defect but are also required to make immediate treatment decisions. Lifelong disability is presumed with this diagnosis. Realities include frequent hospitalizations; concern about life-threatening events; and adjustment of and to a child with a disability.

The mourning process is initiated in each parent with the significant loss of the ideal child. Initial shock is succeeded by the variety of mood states associated with the mourning process. The timing and sequence of grief reactions has not been fully delineated. Kennedy

(1970) suggested that a continuation of the mood state longer than 2 to 3 months is "chronic sorrow." Phillips (1991) also suggested that the certainty and permanence of the disability must be present before chronic sorrow can occur. Regardless of the timing, duration, intensity, and rate of grief, response will vary with each parent (Dyson & Fewell, 1986; Phillips, 1991; Zamerowski, 1982).

Chronic sorrow is, therefore, a recurrent, cyclical emotional response to caring for a child with a disability. The characteristics of this response have variously been described as sadness, hostility, depression, anger, and guilt. Periodic recurrences of grief may affect parental views or perceptions of their child. Mood states, such as chronic sorrow, are thought to affect perception through the cognitive processing component necessary for perceptual accuracy (Forgas & Bower, 1987).

Perceptual accuracy is necessary for accurate parental estimates of their child's development. Studies of parental accuracy in parents of children with neural tube defect have most frequently been with cognitive development. Parents of sick children tend to emphasize normality of development because they like to perceive themselves as coping (McBride, 1984). Sequential accrual of developmental milestones is also expected. Absent or delayed achievement of developmental milestones may occur in children with neural tube defect. Sorrow recurs and reactivates the tendency to emphasize normality regardless of actual performance, resulting in inaccurate perceptions of the child's development. This study, therefore, explored the relationship between chronic sorrow and accuracy of parental perception of the child's cognitive development using King's interacting systems framework (1981) and person perception theory.

King's Systems Framework

King (1981) described individuals as personal systems that interact with other individuals in a variety of transactions or human interactions. Individuals actively process, organize, and categorize experiential and environmental information to provide meaning and stability.

Several concepts form the basis for the personal system, including self, growth and development, and perception. King (1981) defined these concepts in the following ways:

1. Self: This is "a composite of thoughts and feelings which constitute a person's awareness of his [or her] individual existence. . . . includes . . . a system of ideas, attitudes, values and commitments. . . . a person's total subjective environment" (p. 27).
2. Characteristics of growth and development: These are composed of environmental and genetic factors promoting movement to maturity with internal cellular as well as external behavioral changes.
3. Perception: "a process of organizing, interpreting, and transforming information from sensory data and memory. It is a process of human transactions with environment. It gives meaning to one's experience, represents one's image of reality, and influences one's behavior" (p. 24).

In this study, the unit of analysis was the parent. Interest in the accuracy of perception, however, focused on the dyadic relationship of parent and child. Study variables, therefore, included factors of the personal systems of both parent and child.

In the personal system of the parent, the self was represented by the parent and his or her fantasy of the ideal child, an extension of the parent's self. Loss of the ideal child created a change in the parent's mood state and emotional reaction with initiation of the mourning process and chronic sorrow. Growth and development were represented in the child's personal system by focusing on cognitive development. Perception was represented by the accuracy of the parent's image and appraisal of the actual child (Figure 10.1). The dyadic representation of accuracy also focused attention on person perception theory.

Person Perception Theory

Consistent with King's (1981) framework, this study viewed perception as each individual's subjective, personal, and selective "representation of reality" (p. 20). Person perception theory also uses

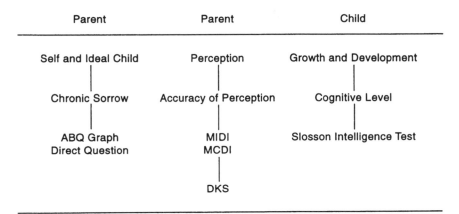

Figure 10.I. Conceptual Theoretical Empirical Framework
NOTE: DKS = Developmental Knowledge Scale; MIDI = Minnesota Infant Developmental Inventory; MCDI = Minnesota Child Developmental Inventory; ABQ = Adapted Burke Questionnaire.

"representations of reality." In this theory, parental cognitive structures are used to organize perception of the child. Their expectations provide internal factors that form the basis for perceptual accuracy. Inference also plays a central role (Wright & Dawson, 1988).

Perception occurs through a variety of processes. Gilbert, Pelham, and Krull (1988) defined three processes for perceivers: categorization, characterization, and correction. Each process requires some cognitive processing. Categorization and characterization appear to occur more reflexively, using few cognitive resources. Correction, however, requires more mental processing (e.g., altering one's first impression of an individual after consideration of their attributes). Person perception is therefore a process by which individuals cognitively make inferences about other individuals and their characteristics.

Many factors may affect person perception. Some arise internally; others come from the environment. In this study, the mood state of chronic sorrow was postulated to affect accuracy of parental perception. Chronic sorrow is the internal, parental factor, initiated as a response to having a child with a neural tube defect.

Ability to work through the grief also requires significant mental processing (Gyulay, 1989). As a result, a parent whose cognitive resources are consumed with sorrow may identify and infer behaviors but be unable to correct characterizations of these behaviors because he or she is "cognitively busy." This process results in inaccurate perceptions. Because both grief and perception use cognitive-mental structures for processing, the cognitive business of sorrow will affect the accuracy of perception. Forgas and Bower (1987) state, "The way a perceiver feels at the time is one of the most important influences in social judgment" (p. 53).

Kruglanski (1989) concluded that determination of perceptual accuracy includes three components: target judgment, criterion, and the correspondence between the two. In this study, accuracy of perception was defined as congruence between the parental assessment of the child and an accepted standard measure. Each component of perception is governed by cognitive and motivational factors. Emphasis is placed on the psychological factors that may affect accuracy.

Kruglanski (1989) defines several categories of the components (e.g., availability of inferential rule, motivation) that are affected by psychological factors that may, in turn, influence the judgment and accuracy process. The judgment in this study was that of cognitive development and the psychological state that of chronic sorrow. Sorrow was measured with choice of adjustment graph, a direct question, and the Adapted Burke Questionnaire. Three measures of chronic sorrow were used to provide comprehensive data about the concept.

Cognitive development was defined as the accrual of mental skills resulting from the interaction of the child with his or her environment. Cognitive development was measured with the Slosson Intelligence Test (SIT). Parental judgment of development was measured by the Minnesota Child Development Inventory (MCDI) and Minnesota Infant Development Inventory (MIDI). Accuracy was then measured by comparing parental responses on the MCDI or MIDI to the SIT.

The scores from the sorrow instruments were correlated to the accuracy score to determine the presence or absence of a relationship. It was postulated that, because mood states affect accuracy and chronic sorrow is a mood state, chronic sorrow affects accuracy.

Parental Differences

In addition, each parent's assessment was considered because mothers and fathers perceive as individuals. Consistent with King (1981), they will have unique transactions with the environment and create their own images of reality. They also have differing past experiences and will view their child's cognitive development with more or less accuracy and congruency. Research in the disabled population has demonstrated differences between mothers and fathers in their coping strategies and styles and coping roles. Schilling, Schinke, and Kirkham (1985) report that women used a combination of cognitive and interpersonal strategies, whereas men use primarily cognitive strategies. In the parents of children with a disability, mothers are more likely than fathers to give meaning to a stressful situation.

Other studies of differences between mothers and fathers or male and female perceptions have occurred in nonparents and parents of disabled children. Additional studies of stress in the disabled population have demonstrated higher distress and/or reported problems in mothers compared to fathers (Goldberg, Marcovitch, MacGregor, & Lojkasek, 1986; Kazak & Marvin, 1984; Tavormina, Boll, Dunn, Luscomb, & Taylor, 1981). Cleve's (1989) study of 100 parents of spina bifida children demonstrated an increase in the coping strategies of crying, busying self with other activities, ignoring the problem, and getting away in mothers compared to fathers ($p = .01$). Studies of adults who are not parents include those conducted by Card, Jackson, Stollack, and Ialongo (1986), who demonstrated that females were more accurate than males on gender-related traits, and by McBride (1985), who demonstrated that women were more extreme than men in their ratings in judgmental situations in which they were confident. Consistent with King's (1981) definition, these studies validate the unique parental perspectives that affect perception.

In summary, perceptual accuracy is affected by mood states. Although both inaccurate perceptions and chronic sorrow have been documented in the parents of disabled children, the relationship between these variables has not been delineated. In addition, mothers and fathers differ in their stress-coping responses to the birth of a child with a disability. Those differences have not yet been identified for the relationship between chronic sorrow and accuracy of perception. The research questions explored in this study, therefore, included that of a relationship between chronic sorrow and accuracy of perception of a child's cognitive development as well as differences in that relationship for mothers and fathers:

1. What is the relationship between chronic sorrow and accuracy of perception of a child's cognitive development in parents of children with neural tube defect?
2. What are the differences between mothers and fathers in the relationship between chronic sorrow and accuracy of perception of a child's cognitive development?

Significance of the Study

One in every thousand live births results in the delivery of a child with myelomeningocele, the most common neural tube defect diagnosed at birth. Although improved medical technology has increased the survival of children with this diagnosis, they require continuous health care and nursing care due to the multiplicity of problems they experience. Nursing care of very young children focuses attention on the parent-child dyad.

Delivery of optimal care to the parent-disabled child dyad requires technical proficiency as well as knowledge of parental factors that influence child care. Parental factors that influence care delivery include accuracy of perception and chronic sorrow. Current research has suggested that both sorrow and inaccurate perceptions are present in the mothers and some fathers of children with a disability (Burke, 1989; Damrosch & Perry, 1989; Keith & Markie, 1969; Tew, Laurence, & Samuel, 1974). Mood states and emotions have been suggested to affect perception. To date, research has focused on the relationship in laboratory settings using undergraduate students.

Current research has also suggested differences between maternal and paternal responses (Russell & Russell, 1982; Schilling et al., 1985). To date, these responses have not been systematically investigated. Specifically lacking are data on paternal responses and parental responses at early developmental stages.

Delineation of the relationship between chronic sorrow and accuracy of perception will provide basic information for parent-focused interventions with these parents. Nursing's goal is to promote health maintenance of individuals for adequate role function (King, 1981). Essential to this goal is an understanding of health. King (1981) described three fundamental health needs of human beings, one of which is presentation of usable information. This information must be presented when it is needed as well as at a time when the individual can use it. A knowledge of the timing of sorrow, an appreciation of the ways it may be manifested, and knowledge to provide information in the face of chronic sorrow will enable the nurse to plan interventions for a time congruent with the parents' response.

Recent legislative change in rights to education for the disabled population (PL 99-457: Individuals With Disability Education Act) has created a clear opportunity for nursing intervention in a variety of areas (Hansen, Holaday, & Miles, 1990). Use of this change is consistent with time as defined by King (1981). She defines time as a sequence of events moving to the future that are influenced by the past.

These interventions may include development of transdisciplinary care, early case finding, and family-oriented educational support. The timing of these interventions is not currently clear. Many factors affect both the children and their parents, and a knowledge of the impact of these factors will be crucial in planning optimal timely intervention. The appearance of chronic sorrow in parents of these children is one such factor that may inhibit parental learning and/or involvement with their disabled children at crucial times. The current study will add to the knowledge base, through use of King's (1981) interacting systems framework, essential information about paternal responses and will clarify the links between chronic sorrow and accuracy of perception in parents of young children.

Summary

Sixty-eight mothers, 64 fathers, and 69 children with neural tube defect participated in the study. The first research question was not supported. Only fathers demonstrated a relationship between chronic sorrow and accuracy of perception. The second research question was supported. There were clear parental differences in both sorrow responses and accuracy of perception. Both chronic sorrow and inaccurate perception were demonstrated in mothers and fathers.

The presence of chronic sorrow and inaccurate perceptions documented in this study supports the presence of components of the personal system in the study parents. In addition, the clear parental differences support the unique, individual representations of reality for each parent. The inability to demonstrate a relationship in all parents between chronic sorrow and accuracy of perception does not permit comment on the potential interactions between components of the personal system.

References

Burke, M. L. (1989). Chronic sorrow in mothers of school-age children with a myelomeningocele disability. *Dissertations Abstracts International, 50,* 233-234B. (University Microfilms No. 89-20 093)

Card, A. L., Jackson, L. A., Stollack, G. E., & Ialongo, N. S. (1986). Gender role and person-perception accuracy. *Sex Roles, 3/4,* 159-171.

Cleve, L. V. (1989). Parental coping response to their child's spina bifida. *Journal of Pediatric Nursing, 4,* 172-176.

Damrosch, S. P., & Perry, L. A. (1989). Self-reported adjustment, chronic sorrow, and coping of parents of children with Down Syndrome. *Nursing Research, 38,* 25-30.

Drotar, D., Baskiewicz, B. A., Irvin, N., Kennell, J., & Klaus, M. (1975). The adaptation of parents to the birth of an infant with a congenital malformation: A hypothetical model. *Pediatrics, 56,* 710-717.

Dyson, L., & Fewell, R. R. (1986). Stress and adaptation in parents of young handicapped and nonhandicapped children: A comparative study. *Journal of the Division for Early Education, 10,* 25-34.

Forgas, J. P., & Bower, G. H. (1987). Mood effects on person-perception judgments. *Journal of Personality and Social Psychology, 53,* 53-60.

Gilbert, D. T., Pelham, B. W., & Krull, D. S. (1988). On cognitive busyness: When person perceivers meet persons perceived. *Journal of Personality and Social Psychology, 54,* 733-740.

Goldberg, S., Marcovitch, S., MacGregor, D., & Lojkasek, M. (1986). Family responses to developmentally delayed preschoolers: Etiology and the father's role. *American Journal of Mental Deficiency, 90,* 610-617.

Gyulay, J. (1989). Grief responses. *Issues in Comprehensive Pediatric Nursing, 12,* 1-31.

Hansen, S., Holaday, B., & Miles, M. S. (1990). The role of the pediatric nurse in a federal program for infants and young children with handicaps. *Journal of Pediatric Nursing, 5,* 246-251.

Kazak, A. E., & Marvin, R. S. (1984). Differences, difficulties and adaptation: Stress and social networks in families with a handicapped child. *Family Relations, 33,* 67-77.

Keith, R. A., & Markie, G. S. (1969). Parental and professional assessment of functioning in cerebral palsy. *Developmental Medicine and Child Neurology, 11,* 735-742.

Kennedy, J. F. (1970). Maternal reactions to the birth of a defective baby. *Social Casework, 51,* 410-416.

King, I. M. (1981). *A theory for nursing: Systems, concepts, process.* New York: Delmar.

Kruglanski, A. W. (1989). The psychology of being "right": The problem of accuracy in social perception and cognition. *Psychological Bulletin, 106,* 395-409.

McBride, A. B. (1984). The experience of being a parent. In H. H. Werley & J. J. Fitzpatrick (Eds.), *Annual Review of Nursing Research* (Vol. 2, pp. 63-81). New York: Springer.

McBride, A. B. (1985). Differences in women's and men's thinking about parent-child interactions. *Research in Nursing and Health, 8,* 389-396.

Phillips, M. (1991). Chronic sorrow in mothers of chronically ill and disabled children. *Issues in Comprehensive Pediatric Nursing, 14,* 111-120.

Russell, A., & Russell, G. (1982). Mother, father, and child beliefs about development. *Journal of Psychology, 110,* 297-306.

Schilling, R. F., Schinke, S. P., & Kirkham, M. A. (1985). Coping with a handicapped child: Differences between mothers and fathers. *Social Science and Medicine, 21,* 857-863.

Solnit, A. J., & Stark, M. H. (1961). Mourning and the birth of a defective child. *Psychoanalytic Study of the Child, 16,* 523-537.

Tavormina, J. B., Boll, N. J., Dunn, R. L., Luscomb, R. L., & Taylor, J. R. (1981). Psychosocial effects on parents of raising a physically handicapped child. *Journal of Abnormal Child Psychology, 9*(1), 121-131.

Tew, B., Laurence, K. M., & Samuel, P. (1974). Parental estimates of the intelligence of their physically handicapped child. *Developmental Medicine and Child Neurology, 16,* 494-500.

Wright, J. C., & Dawson, V. L. (1988). Person perception and the bounded rationality of social judgment. *Journal of Personality and Social Psychology, 55,* 780-794.

Zamerowski, S. T. (1982). Helping families to cope with handicapped children. *Topics in Clinical Nursing, 4,* 41-56.

11

Defining the Health
of a Social System Within
Imogene King's Framework

CHRISTINA L. SIELOFF

Imogene King (1971), within her systems framework, discussed and defined four major concepts of interest to nursing: person, environment, health, and nursing. The goal for nursing was identified as the health of individuals and groups. Although King did not extensively develop the construct of health for groups, her framework provides an opportunity to consider the health of social systems. In 1981, King indicated that, for the health of communities to be measured, the critical attributes of a social system had to be identified.

The purpose of this chapter is to define the health of a social system using a modified process of construct derivation. Constructs that are essential for the successful functioning of a system will be presented and briefly discussed. These constructs will be redefined to identify the critical attributes of the health of a social system.

Relevance of the Health
of a Social System to Nursing

Since 1971, King has included the construct of social system as an essential concept within her systems framework. In 1981, she reinforced this position by identifying social system as a construct that "is essential for a conceptual framework for nursing" (p. 113).

In addition, she identified that the "focus of nursing is the care of human beings" (King, 1981, p. 10). Taken together, these statements direct nurse researchers, theorists, and practitioners to focus on the care of human beings within a social system context. King (1981) also identified that the domain of nursing includes health restoration, maintenance, and promotion. By not identifying a specific system focus for this domain, King provided an opportunity for a health focus to include the health of social systems. Twaddle (1974) further identified the importance of this construct—health of a social system—in stating that health is "a functional requisite of social systems" (p. 31). However, efforts to define the health of a social system have not been published.

Construct Derivation of
the Health of a Social System

Construct derivation is a strategy for construct development in which a construct from one field is transposed to a construct in another field. The transposed construct is then redefined within the second field (Walker & Avant, 1983). Generally, the process of construct derivation consists of an initial review of the literature in an area of interest. As part of the review, the degree to which constructs are developed is analyzed. If it is determined that construct derivation is needed, the literature from other areas is examined to identify a construct that could assist in understanding the substantive area of interest. The selected construct is then redefined within the context of that substantive area (Walker & Avant, 1983).

The process of construct derivation has been modified for this chapter. King's (1981) definition of health for a personal system (an individual) is transposed to health of a social system, another major system within her framework. Dimensions of a successfully functioning system from system literature are proposed as the critical attributes of a healthy system and then redefined within the context of a social system. The transposed definition of health of a social system is as follows: The dynamic experiences of a social system, which implies continuous adjustment to stressors in the internal and external environment through optimum use of the system's resources to achieve maximum potential.

Critical Attributes of the Health of a Social System

In reviewing the literature regarding systems and the attributes that are important for the successful functioning of systems, two major groups of constructs were identified (Anderson & Carter, 1978): constructs that maintain the structure of a system and constructs that facilitate change in a system. Constructs that serve to maintain the structure of the system include openness, self-regulation, and negentropy (negative entropy). Constructs that serve to facilitate change in the structure of the system include differentiation, integration, and goal directedness. Because "systems are always both changing and maintaining themselves at any given time" (Anderson & Carter, 1978, p. 21), both sets of constructs must be present if a social system is to function successfully. Each group of constructs will be briefly described and defined and then redefined within King's (1981) framework.

Attributes That Facilitate the Maintenance of a System

For a system to function successfully, it must be maintained. This is accomplished through the use of openness, self-regulation, and negentropy. Maintenance attributes "help to prevent the system from changing too rapidly and also tend to prevent the various subsystems and the total system from getting out of balance" (Arndt & Huckabay, 1975, p. 36).

Openness involves the processes of input, throughput, and output of information (McFarland, Leonard, & Morris, 1984). To be open is to continuously "exchange matter or energy with the environment" (Hazzard, 1973, p. 179). *Feedback* is an integral component of this processing of information and refers to a "term used to describe the situation in which some portion of a system's output is returned to that system as input in order to modify subsequent outputs of the system" (Pierce, 1973, p. 222). Openness ensures the feedback process that, in turn, aids the maintenance of the system's steady state (Arndt & Huckabay, 1975).

King (1981) states that open systems are characterized by "human beings interacting with their environment . . . [with] continuous and dynamic communication" (p. 66). Through this communication, a social system continuously adjusts to stressors in the internal and external environments. To achieve this adjustment, a social system must be open and receptive to the internal and external environments and must use its feedback mechanism. Openness, therefore, can be redefined as a continuous and dynamic communication system between a system's internal and external environments that is receptive and that effectively uses its feedback mechanisms. This communication system facilitates the social system's adjustment to internal and external stressors, thereby contributing to the social system's health.

The second attribute important for the successful maintenance of a system is *self-regulation*. To self-regulate, a system

> must be capable of detecting any variation between a disturbed state and a normal state. . . . For specific corrective action to be initiated, the variation must be identified and discriminated from other possible variations and the system must be permitted to make the correction for the regulation to be effective. (Hazzard, 1973, p. 181)

Self-regulation is based on the concepts of feedback and *equifinality*. The latter term refers to a situation in which "identical results can be obtained from different initial conditions" (Arndt & Huckabay, 1975, p. 37). Equifinality allows the system to achieve similar outcomes through a variety of means.

Self-regulation is one of the "broad functions of a living system
. . . [and] provides for coping with the internal and external environment" (King, 1975, p. 5). The social system must have mechanisms
in place that provide for the detection of an internal disturbance.
Once disturbances are identified, existing mechanisms within the
social system act to correct the disturbances and monitor the results
of the corrective actions through feedback. Both sets of mechanisms
must be sufficiently flexible to allow for creative approaches to attain
specified outcomes (equifinality).

Self-regulation is also evident in discussions of two constructs
(King, 1981) associated with social systems: organization and decision making. In discussing organization, King (1981) identified that
"growth and viability through feedback" (p. 118) were associated
with organization. Within her discussion related to decision making,
King identified that decisions have a role in "regulat[ing] each person's life and work" (p. 132); decision making is continuous with
one decision leading to others. Drawing from the literature cited,
self-regulation can be redefined as the creative mechanisms that
(a) efficiently identify disturbance in a social system, (b) use effective
decision-making processes, and (c) institute timely corrective activities that are monitored through effective feedback mechanisms.
These self-regulation mechanisms facilitate the social system's adjustment to internal and external stressors, thereby contributing to
the social system's health.

Negentropy is the third attribute required for the successful maintenance of a system. Negentropy, or negative entropy, is achieved
through system processes that decrease the energy within a system
that is not usable (Bertrand, 1972; Hazzard, 1973). A system must
maintain energy within itself to accomplish the work of the system.
If a system moves "toward an unorganized state characterized by
decreased interactions among its components" (Anderson & Carter,
1978, p. 15), there will be a decrease in the energy that can be used.

Although King (1981) does not directly address negentropy, the
concepts identified as important for understanding social systems
could be viewed as regulators of energy use. For example, she states
that "standards or norms based on a set of roles and status" (p. 22)
serve to direct interactions of social members. Facilitating social
system interactions would decrease the energy needed for those

interactions. In further clarifying the concept of authority, King (1981) identified that it "provides order . . . [and] guides and directs behavior" (p. 123). Clearly defined lines of authority also decrease the energy needed by the social system through the provision of order and direction for behavior. In addition, King identified power as "analogous to energy in the physical world [and] . . . essential in an organization for the maintenance of balance and harmony" (p. 126). A "misuse of power may cause chaos and disorganization" (p. 127). Hence a positive use of power could be seen to increase organization and, therefore, be negentropic.

By providing a structure for the work of the social system, standards, norms, authority, and power serve to decrease the amount of energy required by a system to conduct its routine functioning. By reducing the amount of energy required by a social system, these concepts increase the amount of energy available for work. It follows that standards and norms, clearly defined lines of authority, and effective use of power define the negentropy in the social system. Taken together, these attributes decrease the energy needed for routine functioning of the social system, thereby optimizing the use of the system's energy, its major resource.

Attributes That Facilitate Change in a System

It is also important for a system to change if it is to function successfully. The attributes that have been identified as facilitating change in a system include differentiation, integration, and goal directedness.

In the process of *differentiation*, there is "further development, specialization, and elaboration within a clearly perceived system" (Bowler, 1981, p. 153). Created from the process of differentiation, subsystems evolve as a result of "perceived stress" (Bowler, 1981, p. 154) to the system and focus on the accomplishment of something that needs to be done. Differentiation can also be demonstrated through "progressive segregation. This process occurs when the system subdivides into a hierarchical order of subordinate systems that gain some degree of independence of each other" (Arndt & Huckabay, 1975, p. 35). Through this differentiation, organization is achieved.

Within a social system, subsystems would develop on the basis of the specialized skills and knowledge needed to enable a social system to cope with stressors while achieving its tasks. Within King's (1971) systems framework, the constructs of authority, roles, and status aid in the development of specialized subsystems designed to assist a social system to cope with stressors. Each of these constructs could also serve to organize subsystems within the original social system.

King (1981) further discussed differentiation in relation to her constructs of organization and status. A structural characteristic of organization is the "formal and informal arrangements of . . . groups to achieve individual and organizational goals" (p. 117). Differentiation of groups occurs in order for goals to be achieved. Once these arrangements exist, status contributes to the "position of . . . a group in relation to other groups in an organization" (p. 129), which could lead to further differentiation. The concept of differentiation is redefined as the formal and informal arrangements of groups, based on specialized knowledge and skills, which are directed toward the achievement of goals. These arrangements of groups promote the optimum use of a social system's resources, thereby contributing to the social system's health.

"For a system to survive, what has been differentiated must be integrated" (Bowler, 1981, p. 158). *Integration* involves the coordination of the various functions of the subsystems that have been created (Pierce, 1973). Without such coordination, system energy would be wasted through duplication or counterproductive efforts. For a social system to survive, what has been differentiated into subsystems must then be integrated through appropriate mechanisms. Although King (1981) does not specifically address integration, her discussion of the construct of organization identifies the importance of the "interrelationships of units to accomplish goals" (p. 118). Interrelationships of subsystems must be fostered if a social system is to accomplish its goals most effectively. Accordingly, the concept of integration is redefined as mechanisms that foster the interrelationships of subsystems to achieve goals. These interrelationships promote the optimum use of resources by decreasing duplication of efforts, thereby contributing to the social system's health.

Goal directedness is the third characteristic that facilitates change in a system. The "measure of the effectiveness of [a system] is its capacity to enable the fulfillment of the system's goals as well as the goals of the component elements of the system" (Anderson & Carter, 1978, p. 20). The system's organization and functioning must facilitate the attainment of the goals by the system and its component parts.

King (1975) stated that "one of the properties of a living system . . . is that behavior is goal-directed" (p. 5). Goal directedness permeates the concepts identified as relevant to social systems. According to King (1981), organization is an "environment in which resources are available to achieve goals . . . [and is] characterized by structure, function and resources to achieve goals" (p. 116). Authority is "essential to the achievement of goals . . . [and is] used to coordinate and regulate behaviors to achieve goals" (p. 123). Power is *goal-directed* [italics added]. . . . If there are no goals, there is no power" (p. 127). "Decisions are *goal-directed* [italics added] . . . [with the] effectiveness of decisions [being] evaluated in terms of goal attainment" (pp. 132-133). The concept of goal directedness is redefined as (a) clearly defined goals, (b) resources that are directed toward the achievement of goals, (c) authority that is used to "coordinate and regulate behaviors to achieve goals" (King, 1981, p. 123), (d) effective use of power, and (e) a decision-making process that is goal directed and evaluated in terms of the attainment of goals. These attributes focus the social system's activities on the attainment of goals, contributing to the achievement of its potential and health.

In summary, critical attributes that indicate the health of a social system include the following:

1. Continuous and dynamic communication between the system's internal and external environments, receptivity, and effective feedback mechanisms (openness)
2. Mechanisms that efficiently identify disturbance in the system, effective decision-making processes, timely corrective mechanisms that are monitored through effective feedback mechanisms, and creativity (self-regulation)
3. Standards and norms, clearly defined lines of authority, and the effective use of power (negentropy)
4. Formal and informal arrangement of groups, based on specialized knowledge and skills, directed toward the achievement of goals (differentiation)

5. Mechanisms fostering the interrelationships of subsystems to achieve goals (integration)
6. Clearly defined goals, resources directed toward the achievement of goals, authority that is used to "coordinate and regulate behaviors to achieve goals" (King, 1981, p. 123), effective use of power, a decision-making process that is goal directed and evaluated in terms of the attainment of goals (goal directedness).

Directions for Research

Research related to the health of a social system could take several approaches: (a) operationally defining the health of a social system; (b) defining the health of specific social systems, such as a nursing department, using the identified attributes; and (c) instrument development designed to estimate the health of a social system in general or a specific social system, such as a nursing department. Research questions, investigating relationships between the identified attributes to determine that attributes explain the largest portion of the health variance, might include the following:

1. Must all six variables be present for a social system to demonstrate health?
2. Which variable contributes to the largest proportion of the variance of health?
3. How are the six variables related to each other?

This type of research would contribute to the development of nursing theory regarding social systems within King's (1981) systems framework. Such nursing theory would assist nurse administrators by providing a theory base for their practice that is founded within nursing rather than within business administration.

Summary

The development of a definition of the health of a social system originated within the framework of Imogene King, a recognized nurse theorist. Although King (1981) discussed the concept of health primarily in relation to the personal system, her framework provides an opportunity to consider the health of both interpersonal and social systems. It is important to examine health from a social systems perspective because health indicates optimal functioning, and optimal functioning is (a) important for all systems and (b) an identified goal of nursing.

References

Anderson, R. E., & Carter, I. (1978). *Human behavior in the social environment: A social systems approach.* New York: Aldine.

Arndt, C., & Huckabay, L. M. D. (1975). *Nursing administration: Theory for practice with a systems approach.* St. Louis, MO: C. V. Mosby.

Bertrand, A. L. (1972). *Social organization: A general systems and role theory perspective.* Philadelphia: F. A. Davis.

Bowler, T. D. (1981). *General systems thinking: Its scope and applicability.* New York: North Holland.

Hazzard, M. E. (1973). An overview of system theory. In M. E. Hardy (Ed.), *Theoretical foundations for nursing* (pp. 176-184). New York: MSS Information.

King, I. M. (1971). *Toward a theory for nursing: General concepts of human behavior.* New York: John Wiley.

King, I. M. (1975). Patient aspects. In L. J. Shuman, R. Dixon Speas, Jr., & J. P. Young (Eds.), *Operations research in health care: A critical analysis* (pp. 3-20). Baltimore: The Johns Hopkins University Press.

King, I. M. (1981). *A theory for nursing: Systems, concepts, process.* New York: John Wiley.

McFarland, G. K., Leonard, H. S., & Morris, M. M. (1984). *Nursing leadership and management: Contemporary strategies.* New York: John Wiley.

Pierce, L. M. (1973). Usefulness of a systems approach for problem conceptualization and investigation. In M. E. Hardy (Ed.), *Theoretical foundations for nursing* (pp. 217-226). New York: MSS Information.

Twaddle, A. C. (1974). The concept of health status. *Social Science Medicine,* 8(1), 29-38.

Walker, L. O., & Avant, K. C. (1983). *Strategies for theory construction in nursing.* Norwalk, CT: Appleton-Century-Crofts.

12

Using Health, Personal, and Interpersonal System Concepts Within King's Systems Framework to Explore Perceived Health Status During the Menopause Transition

NANCY C. SHARTS-HOPKO

At the time this study was designed, menopause was still a little studied but much dreaded phenomenon (Feeley & Pyne, 1975; LaRocco & Polit, 1980). It was described as the only natural event still to be called a disease and the last to be researched (Rothman, 1989). One of the most compelling attractions of women's experience of menopause was the marked contrast between transcultural studies, which often described positive or neutral associations with menopause (Flint, 1975; Kaufert, 1980; Skultans, 1970; Wright, 1980), and American studies, which documented negative expectations about aging in general, aging in women, and menopause in particular (Bart,

1972; Wilbush, 1981). Menopause was overwhelmingly portrayed in the medical, psychoanalytic, and lay literature as a hormone deficiency disease requiring medical treatment (Campbell & Whitehead, 1977; Dennerstein, Burrows, Hyman, & Sharpe, 1979; Leppert, 1981).

This study, drawing on the conceptualization of health and of personal and interpersonal systems within the King (1981) systems framework, sought to explore factors related to midlife women's perceived health status throughout the menopause transition. Specifically, the study addressed the relationships between menopausal stage, current life change, attitude toward women's roles, menopausal symptoms, use of hormone therapy, socioeconomic status, and perceived health status among women ages 40 through 55 (Sharts Engel, 1984, 1987). Other previously unreported factors emerging from the review of literature were explored, including perception of one's mother's menopause experience, perception of one's life partner's attitude toward menopause, and the perceived timing of menopause (Dosey & Dosey, 1980; Neugarten, 1979; Uphold & Susman, 1981; Woods, 1980).

King's Systems Framework and Women's Experience of Menopause

King's (1981) systems framework clearly and concisely expresses assumptions and beliefs underlying this investigation. Within the framework, individuals are viewed as open systems interacting within a cultural context. Concepts within the framework used to describe individuals of particular relevance to this study include perception, self, growth and development, and time. Concepts used to describe persons in interactions that are particularly relevant to this study include role and stress.

Individuals, or personal systems, are described as ever diversifying, unified, and in continual interaction with their internal and external environments. Individuals perceive, or have awareness of, a representation of reality from their own unique perspectives. Self is a dynamic internal construct of one's experience of others and of the environment. Personal systems are characterized by growth and development, a unidirectional flow of events through the life process. Such change is influenced by genetic endowment, experience, and the environment. Time, or the way people perceive the succession of events in their lives, is measurable but also subjective. Personal systems exist in relationship to other individuals and social systems; various roles are fulfilled. Role is a situational set of learned behaviors played out in interaction with others. Role is dynamic and reciprocal. King (1981) views perception of self as influenced by role and role expectations of others. Individuals are characterized by greater or lesser degrees of stress, a dynamic, individual, personal, and subjective state that describes energy exchange between the personal system and the environments, both internal and external.

King (1981) describes health as the way individuals deal with the stresses of growth and development while functioning within their cultural context. Menopause is one developmental process occurring among women in middle adulthood. It reflects a change in the internal environment. The experience of menopause may demand reformulation of a woman's view of herself. Self-evaluation occurs against a backdrop of learned or perceived social standards.

Within American society, the menopause transition has been the subject of fear and myth, although there is still no clear evidence that menopause is inherently debilitating for most women. Several prior studies suggest that as the unknown becomes known and women experience menopause for themselves, their view of it improves (Kaufert, 1980; Neugarten, Wood, Kraines, & Loomis, 1963). Therefore, it was hypothesized that the later the menopausal stage, from premenopause through perimenopause into postmenopause, the more positively women would view their health.

Women do experience menopause within a cultural and interpersonal context. It is likely that concurrent upheaval in their lives will be negatively related to how they experience menopause. Within King's (1981) framework, stress is viewed as an individual's energy response to elements in the environment that have the capacity to alter perception of reality. The utility of this notion in considering the menopause experience is supported by previous studies. Skultans (1970) observed that Welsh village women were more likely to complain about menopause if they also experienced marital and sexual difficulties. The observations of Uphold and Susman (1981) and others (Ballinger, 1975; Cooke & Greene, 1981) that the occurrence of menopausal symptoms is positively related to family stress lend support to the hypothesis that current life change is negatively associated with perceived health status in menopausal women.

In addition, women's experience of menopause may be heavily influenced by the extent to which they are invested in the childbearing and child-rearing role. Transcultural research has supported this view with observations that release from menstrual taboos is associated with the absence of a menopausal syndrome (Flint, 1975; Wright, 1980). Bart (1972) noted that more passive and traditional American women were more likely to be hospitalized for depression at menopause than less traditional, more outgoing women. These studies lend support to the hypothesis that nontraditional attitudes toward women's roles are positively related to perceived health status among menopausal women.

Tallying of menopausal symptoms has proved inadequate to explain women's experience of menopause and their perception of self (Dosey & Dosey, 1980; Neugarten et al., 1963; Skultans, 1970). From the review of literature, what seems more important is a woman's expectation of when menopause will occur, her perception of her own health, her help-seeking behavior, and other aspects of her feminine identity. Some of this meaning is likely learned from significant others, such as one's mother or life partner.

The relationships of influencing factors on perceived health status are neither sequential nor discrete. For after all, personal systems are unified. Furthermore, menopause as a transition can both generate life stress and be influenced by other concurrent life events. It exemplifies a developmental process characterized by interaction between the personal system and the internal and external environments.

To view the menopause experience as a developmental process, influenced by change in the internal and external environments, women's expectations of menopause, and such social factors as attitude toward women's roles and the perceptions of significant others, is congruent with King's (1981) systems framework. The framework supports the exploration of relationships between these factors and midlife women's perceived health status and help-seeking behavior.

Method

Sample

This study has been previously described in the nursing literature (Sharts Engel, 1984, 1987). Two hundred and forty-nine women between the ages of 40 and 55 were recruited from professional, community, and religious groups. Institutional procedures for the protection of human subjects were followed. Women were not told that this was a study of menopause per se. Rather, it was presented as a study of adult development. Women were excluded from the sample if they experienced mastectomy, hysterectomy, oophorectomy or artificial menopause, or prior mental illness; if they were ill or disabled; if they were pregnant or postpartal at the time of the study; if they had not completed the eighth grade; or if they were not native-born Americans. Presumably these were well American women who were experiencing a natural transition.

The sample was 96% Caucasian, with a mean age of 47.0 years ($SD = 5.46$), a mean level of education of 14.48 years ($SD = 2.62$), and a mean family income of $46,716 per year ($SD = 35,676$). One hundred and eighty-five women were employed outside the home, and another 22 were students or actively involved in volunteer work. In this sample, 215 women had never seen a physician for menopause-related concerns, and only 19 women had ever taken medication for menopause-related problems. None of these factors was significantly related to menopausal stage. There were 83 women, representing each menopausal stage.

Instruments

Menopausal stage was determined by self-report of change in the menstrual cycle. Menopause is viewed as a progression of stages. Premenopause is the time before midlife change in the quality or frequency of menstruation. Perimenopause is the time from onset of menstrual change until 12 months after the last menstrual period. Postmenopause is the time after menses has ceased for 12 months (Metcalf, 1979). In the menopause literature it is a persistent problem that all of the decades after menopause are viewed as a single life stage—postmenopause. In this study, the end point of 55 years was established because it is two standard deviations above the mean age of menopause in North America—49 years.

The Life Experiences Survey (LES) (Sarason, Johnson, & Siegel, 1978) was used to measure current life change. This variation on the Schedule of Recent Events (Holmes & Rahe, 1967) allowed for a desirability and impact rating of each event that had occurred.

The Index of Sex Role Orientation (ISRO) (Dreyer, Woods, & James, 1981) was used to measure attitude toward women's roles, based on value of self primarily as an individual versus value of self primarily as wife, mother, and homemaker.

The Menopause Symptom Checklist (MSC) has frequently been used in the study of middle-aged women despite its questionable validity (Neugarten & Kraines, 1965). Yet the tool's authors demonstrated that the only symptom significantly more common among menopausal women than women of other age groups was hot flashes. This instrument was included in this study precisely because of the issue of its validity.

Perceived Health Status (PHS) was measured by an author-generated instrument that combined existing tools. The Health Perceptions Questionnaire (Ware, 1976) primarily addresses physical health. The Affect Balance Scale (Bradburn, 1969) addresses psychological well-being. And the Life Satisfaction Index (Campbell, Converse, & Rodgers, 1976) assesses social well-being. King (1981) identified the difficulty in measuring health, noting that most measures of health have, in fact, looked at illness. The combination of these three instruments reflected the World Health Organization's definition of health as a "state of complete physical, mental, and social well-being and not merely the absence of disease or infirmity" (Antonovsky, 1980), which acknowledges health's multidimensional nature. At the very least, the PHS tool is in need of refinement (Sharts Engel, 1984). In fact, the struggle to define and measure health continues and is both reflected in and influenced by the ongoing health policy debate on exactly what health and illness care should be guaranteed for the United States' citizenry. All other factors under investigation were assessed using a personal data form.

Analysis included Pearson product moment correlations between all variables and hierarchical regression analysis to determine how much of the variance in PHS score could be accounted for. Age was included as a control variable (Ware, 1976).

Results

The hierarchical regression of factors onto PHS is described. Age, a control variable, was not significant.

Menopausal stage was significantly but inversely related to perceived health status. It accounted for under 2% of variance ($F = 4.53$, $p = .03$, df 1, 246).

The relationship between LES and PHS was significant and in the direction hypothesized, although it accounted for just 2% of variance ($F = 5.29$, $p = .022$, df 1, 245). Interestingly, when positive LES and negative LES scores were regressed separately, they accounted for 2% and 11% of variance, respectively.

When ISRO was entered into the regression, change in R^2 was not significant. But the relationship was curvilinear. When $ISRO^2$ was added, an additional 2% of variance was accounted for ($F = 4.16$, $p = .042$, df 1, 243). A cross-product vector of LES × ISRO accounted for another 3% of variance ($F = 7.89$, $p = .005$, df 1, 242), indicating an interaction effect between those variables.

Menopausal Symptom Checklist score contributed 24.1% of variance ($F = 86.41$, $p < .0001$, df 1, 241), strongly suggesting a relationship between occurrence of symptomatology and the way health is evaluated by these women. Only 1.2% of the sample indicated that they found hot flashes severe and worrisome in the past year. Other symptoms present in over half of the women during the previous year were not associated with any particular menopausal stage.

Perception of mother's menopause experience added 4% to explained variance in PHS ($F = 9.154$, $p < .003$, df 1, 223). Perception of life partner's attitude toward menopause contributed an additional 9% of variance accounted for ($F = 23.43$, $p < .0001$, df 1, 214). The Pearson correlational coefficient for educational level and PHS equaled .14 ($p = .015$, $N = 249$). When hierarchically regressed after the preceding variables, its contribution was not significant. Finally, when perceived timing of menopause (early, on-time, late) was dummy coded as "on-time" or "off-time" and entered into the regression, R^2 equaled .09 ($F = 5.58$, $p < .01$, df 2, 108).

When all variables demonstrating a significant relationship with PHS were regressed after age, R^2 equaled .430 (df 13, 235) when mean substitution was employed; when cases with missing data were deleted, R^2 equaled .51 (df 13, 81). (The difference in Ns reflected the wording of an item stem, "If you are in menopause or the change of life now, or if you have finished with it.")

Discussion

King's (1981) systems framework contributes to this research a way to organize and evaluate a substantial body of literature about menopause reflecting the worldviews of medicine, psychoanalytic thought, anthropology, sociology, and the newly emergent feminist scholarship. King herself drew from multiple disciplines in formulating a nursing view of how health is nurtured among people in their environments. She was well aware of the insufficiency of a medical view of health as the absence of illness or abnormality and of the need to consider how people live and experience their lives. A view of menopause as a normal developmental process that has individual meaning for women reflecting their experiences of their internal and external environments, over time, is in keeping with King's (1981) view of growth and development as "a function of genetic endowment, meaningful and satisfying experiences, and an environment conducive to helping individuals move toward maturity" (p. 31).

The results of this study lend support to the relevance of various social and perceptual factors to the perceived health status of women at various stages of the menopause transition. These factors include current life change, perception of one's mother's experience of menopause, perception of one's life partner's attitude toward menopause, the experience of menopausal symptoms, perceived timing of menopause, and educational level. When all factors were considered together, at least 43% of variance in perceived health status was accounted for. In attitude research, this is substantial.

These results support a view of menopause as suggested by King's (1981) framework. Clearly, a woman's perceived health status during menopause arises from her experience of a changing internal environment, characterized by more or less menopausal symptomatology as well as interaction with her external environment, including current life change and input from significant others concerning the issue of menopause.

The large variance in perceived health status accounted for by menopausal symptomatology was surprising in light of transcultural research that demonstrates little or no relationship between menopause and the experience of symptoms. This finding may be viewed in at least two ways. Women may define health as the absence of symptoms or discomforts and, thus, cognitively interpret the presence of symptoms as indicative of diminished health or aging. Alternatively, they may actually be discomforted by the presence of symptoms. Transcultural research lends support to the former position, and this is consistent with the importance that King (1981) ascribes to personal meaning in defining health.

This study lends some support to a view of menopause as, in part, a learned behavior. Women for whom menopause occurred at the time it was expected more positively perceived their health status than did women who felt that the timing was off. The importance of one's mother's menopause experience can be interpreted as (a) role modeling for how one "does" menopause, (b) evidence for the importance of transactions between individuals in ascribing meaning to developmental processes, (c) support for the perspective that menstrual patterns are a familial trait, or (d) some combination thereof. King's (1981) definition of growth and development allows for all of these interpretations. Further consideration of a learned component as to how menopause is experienced is justified by examining how expectations of pregnancy have evolved in American society over the past three decades.

The significance of perception of one's life partner's attitude toward menopause speaks to an interaction, within the holistic personal system, between perception and self. Part of one's subjective definition of self arises through perception of others' definitions of oneself. This conceptualization is clearly stated in King's (1981) definition of self.

By the time this study was conducted, in the early 1980s, American culture had been changed markedly by the women's movement.

The expectations placed on midlife women, and those that they themselves held, reflected norms that were different from those that had prevailed in the previous generation. Although these were affluent, well-educated Caucasian women, this was not a sample of housewives; less than 20% of these women were primarily home based. Although the relative socioeconomic privilege enjoyed by these women certainly buffers their lives, it can be safely presumed that demographically similar samples have been used in most of the menopause research to date. What has changed over the decades that menopause has been studied is women's movement outside their homes. The high level of perceived well-being and the small contribution of menopausal stage to variance in perceived health status observed in this sample may have reflected the outward focus in their lives and the greater complexity of roles they assumed. King's (1981) framework allows for a continually changing sociocultural milieu.

Although over 40% of variance in perceived health status was accounted for in this study, more than 50% was not. As noted previously (Sharts Engel, 1987), alternative methodologies would likely have better captured the meaning of menopause in women's lives, particularly if a group were to be followed throughout the entire menopause transition. Research in women's health in general has reflected challenge to and transcendence of existing theoretical paradigms and a dissatisfaction with mechanistic research methodologies over the past decade.

To consider just three studies that add considerably to the findings of this one, Woods et al. (1988) turned to 528 women aged 18 to 45 for an answer to the single question, "What does being healthy mean to you?" The health images that emerged reflected a strong emphasis on actualization or well-being, not merely the absence of symptoms, role performance, or adaptation. It would be interesting to pose this question to women aged 40 to 55 to see if the health images carry through the next decade of life.

Wilbur and Dan (1989) have challenged the adequacy of two common perspectives on women's psychological well-being in midlife— the hormonal insufficiency model versus the "empty-nest syndrome" model—with their study of factors associated with psychological well-being among midlife employed nurses. One of their major contributions is the realization that women may experience decreased life satisfaction during a life transition without becoming clinically depressed. This represents a refinement in thinking about individuals' response to life stress and developmental transitions.

Dickson (1990a, 1990b) examined the language of menopause in the medical literature from the 19th century to the present and contrasted this view with the lived experience of menopause shared by 11 women. One of her contributions is increased understanding of the interplay between edicts from the scientific community and women's lived experiences. Women do not experience menopause in a vacuum. This is consistent with the transcultural literature. A number of recent nursing dissertations, including Dickson's (1990a, 1990b), have described qualitative studies of women's experience of menopause in the United States and elsewhere.

Although none of these studies drew from King's (1981) systems framework per se, each is consistent with her view of a unified human system developing through time and perceiving and experiencing situations within the context of dynamic internal and external environments.

Unfortunately, the medical literature as well as the popular lay press continue successfully to promote a view of menopause as deficiency disease that can and should be treated (Manson et al., 1992; Riggs & Melton, 1992; Sheehy, 1992; Stampfer et al., 1991). The challenge for nursing scholarship includes continued work to document fully the range of normal menopause experience for diverse groups of women in this and other cultures, as well as their self-care strategies, their health needs, and their decision making about and responses to hormonal and other medical therapies. In general, nursing scholarship must further efforts to define and measure health and to characterize growth and development throughout adulthood among women and men. The imperative to support individuals in their life situations is a thread running through theory development in nursing from Nightingale to the present. This legacy reflects a vision different from that of medicine's traditional, mechanistic model of pathology and cure. Nursing conceptual frameworks and theories, such as King's (1981), promote the study of individuals' experiences that affect their health, on their own terms, as well as strategies for best supporting individuals through these experiences.

King's framework was last reformulated in 1981. No longer is the concept of individuals as open systems seen as radical, as it was when she began her theoretical work. The way the model's foundational concepts are understood will no doubt evolve as nursing scholarship develops. For example, consider the evolution of standards of health as cultures evolve. Still, as a structure for the integration of knowledge about menopause and about human development in general, the strength of King's systems framework lies in its breadth and its timelessness.

References

Antonovsky, A. (1980). *Health, stress, and coping.* San Francisco: Jossey-Bass.

Ballinger, C. B. (1975). Psychiatric morbidity and the menopause: Screening of general population sample. *British Medical Journal, 3,* 344-346.

Bart, P. (1972). Depression in middle-aged women. In J. M. Bardwick (Ed.), *Readings on the psychology of women* (pp. 134-142). New York: Harper & Row.

Bradburn, N. M. (1969). *The structure of psychological well-being.* Chicago: Aldine.

Campbell, A., Converse, P. E., & Rodgers, W. L. (1976). *The quality of American life: Perceptions, evaluations, satisfactions.* New York: Russell Sage.

Campbell, S., & Whitehead, M. (1977). Oestrogen therapy and the menopausal syndrome. *Clinics in Obstetrics and Gynecology, 4*(1), 31-47.

Cooke, D. J., & Greene, J. G. (1981). Type of life events in relation to symptoms at the climacterium. *Journal of Psychosomatic Research, 25*(1), 5-11.

Dennerstein, L., Burrows, G. D., Hyman, G. J., & Sharpe, K. (1979). Hormone therapy and affect. *Maturitas, 1,* 247-259.

Dickson, G. L. (1990a). A feminist poststructuralist analysis of the knowledge of menopause. *Advances in Nursing Science, 12*(3), 15-31.

Dickson, G. L. (1990b). The metalanguage of menopause research. *Image: Journal of Nursing Scholarship, 22*(3), 168-173.

Dosey, M. F., & Dosey, M. A. (1980). The climacteric woman. *Patient Counselling and Health Education, 2*(1), 14-21.

Dreyer, N. A., Woods, N. F., & James, S. A. (1981). ISRO: A scale to measure sex-role orientation. *Sex Roles, 7*(2), 173-182.

Feeley, E., & Pyne, H. (1975). The menopause: Facts and misconceptions. *Nursing Forum, 14*(1), 74-86.

Flint, M. (1975). The menopause: Reward or punishment? *Psychosomatics, 16*(4), 161-163.

Holmes, T. H., & Rahe, R. H. (1967). The social readjustment rating scale. *Journal of Psychosomatic Research, 11*, 213-218.

Kaufert, P. A. (1980). The perimenopausal woman and her use of health services. *Maturitas, 2*, 191-205.

King, I. (1981). *A theory for nursing: Systems, concepts, process.* New York: John Wiley.

LaRocco, S. A., & Polit, D. F. (1980). Women's knowledge about the menopause. *Nursing Research, 29*(1), 10-13.

Leppert, P. (1981, September). Doctor, will menopause really change my life? *Ladies' Home Journal,* pp. 40-42.

Manson, J. E., Tosteson, H., Ridker, P. M., Satterfield, S., Herbert, P., O'Connor, G. T., Buring, J. E., & Hennekens, C. H. (1992). The primary prevention of myocardial infarction. *New England Journal of Medicine, 326*(21), 1406-1416.

Metcalf, M. G. (1979). Incidence of ovulatory cycles in women approaching the menopause. *Journal of Biosocial Science, 11*(1), 39-48.

Neugarten, B. L. (1979). Time, age and the life cycle. *American Journal of Psychiatry, 136*(7), 887-894.

Neugarten, B. L., & Kraines, R. J. (1965). Menopausal symptoms in women of various ages. *Psychosomatic Medicine, 27*(3), 266-273.

Neugarten, B. L., Wood, V., Kraines, R. J., & Loomis, B. (1963). Women's attitudes toward the menopause. *Vita Humana, 6*, 140-151.

Riggs, B. L., & Melton, L. J. (1992). The prevention and treatment of osteoporosis. *New England Journal of Medicine, 327*(9), 620-627.

Rothman, B. K. (1989). Women, health, and medicine. In J. Freeman (Ed.), *Women: A feminist perspective* (4th ed., pp. 76-86). Mountain View, CA: Mayfield.

Sarason, I. G., Johnson, J. H., & Siegel, J. M. (1978). Assessing the impact of life changes: Development of the life experiences survey. *Journal of Consulting and Clinical Psychology, 46*(3), 932-946.

Sharts Engel, N. (1984). On the vicissitudes of health appraisal. *Advances in Nursing Science, 7*(1), 12-23.

Sharts Engel, N. (1987). Menopausal stage, current life change, attitude toward women's roles and perceived health status among 40- to 55-year-old women. *Nursing Research, 36*(6), 353-357.

Sheehy, G. (1992). *The silent passage: Menopause.* New York: Random House.

Skultans, V. (1970). The symbolic significance of menstruation and the menopause. *Man, 5*(4), 639-651.

Stampfer, M. J., Colditz, G. A., Willett, W. C., Manson, J. E., Rosner, B., Speizer, F. E., & Hennekens, C. H. (1991). Postmenopausal estrogen therapy and cardiovascular disease: Ten year follow-up from the Nurses' Health Study. *New England Journal of Medicine, 325*(11), 756-762.

Uphold, C. R., & Susman, E. J. (1981). Self-reported climacteric symptoms as a function of the relationship between marital adjustment and child-rearing stage. *Nursing Research, 30*(2), 84-88.

Ware, J. E. (1976). Scales for measuring general health perceptions. *Health Services Research, 11*(4), 396-415.

Wilbur, J., & Dan, A. J. (1989). The impact of work patterns on psychological well-being of midlife nurses. *Western Journal of Nursing Research, 11*(6), 703-716.

Wilbush, J. (1981). What's in a name? Some linguistic aspects of the climacteric. *Maturitas, 3*(1), 1-9.

Woods, N. F. (1980). Women's roles and illness episodes: A prospective study. *Research in Nursing and Health, 3,* 137-145.

Woods, N. F., Laffrey, S., Duffy, M., Lentz, M. J., Mitchell, E. S., Taylor, D., & Cowan, K. A. (1988). Being healthy: Women's images. *Advances in Nursing Science, 11*(1), 36-46.

Wright, A. L. (1980). Cultural variability in the experience of menopause: A comparison of Navajo and Western data (Doctoral dissertation, University of Arizona, 1980). *Dissertation Abstracts International, 40,* 592A. (University Microfilms No. 80-11, 128)

13

Implementing Nursing Diagnoses Within the Context of King's Conceptual Framework

ESTHER COKER

THELMA FRADLEY

JANET HARRIS

DIANNE TOMARCHIO

VIVIAN CHAN

CHARMAINE CARON

Conceptual frameworks for nursing and nursing diagnoses are generally acknowledged to hold immense promise for the further development of nursing's scientific base. To date, the nursing profession has failed to link the two, thus diminishing their impact. This

NOTE: Reprinted from *Nursing Diagnosis* with permission from NANDA. *Nursing Diagnosis*, 1, pp. 107-114, 1990.

chapter describes a project undertaken at a 650-bed community hospital in suburban Toronto, Ontario, Canada, to link the North American Nursing Diagnosis Association (NANDA) list of nursing diagnoses with Imogene King's conceptual framework (King, 1981). The hospital's Department of Nursing chose a conceptual framework after careful examination of the values and beliefs of its nurses at all levels. The conceptual framework of Imogene King (1981) was selected as having an assumptive base congruent with the values of the nurses.

The plan for implementation of the framework involved working through the steps of the nursing process. The Nursing Practice Committee, a subcommittee of the Nursing Quality Assurance Committee comprised of 13 nurses from administration, education, and general staff, began by creating the prototype of a nursing history and assessment record. The assessment tool would be modified by specific clinical areas to suit their needs and serve as a guide to help nurses collect data according to King's framework.

Implementation of King's framework was the next challenge. Although the nursing staff seemed to value the use of care plans in practice, they were having difficulty articulating areas of nursing concern that had been identified during the assessment. The Nursing Practice Committee agreed that the problems or areas of concern should be expressed as nursing diagnoses but were concerned that the use of the NANDA list of nursing diagnoses would be viewed by nurses as an exercise removed from the use of King's conceptual framework since no practical tie between the NANDA list of diagnostic categories and a specific theorist exists (Martin & Frank, 1989).

The committee reasoned that a fundamental purpose of a conceptual framework is to direct the collection of data on the basis of a view of the patient, the nurse and patient environment, the purpose of nursing, and the focus of nursing's concern. During history taking, critical defining characteristics of specific nursing diagnoses may emerge from a patient's statements or nonverbal cues. By tying NANDA's nursing diagnoses to the concepts and systems of King's conceptual framework, nurses could be guided in gathering data, clustering defining characteristics, and making clinical inferences based on the nature and organization of the data.

Stage 1:
Development of the Nursing
Diagnoses Categorization Tool

To this end the Nursing Practice Committee began a process of developing a nursing diagnoses categorization tool based on the systems and concepts in the conceptual framework of Imogene King.

Background

King (1981) describes nursing practice as taking place within three dynamic, interacting systems. These systems are made up of concepts that are of interest to nurses. King's *personal system* is comprised of the concepts of perception, self, body image, growth and development, time, and space; the *interpersonal system* encompasses the concepts of interaction, communication, transaction, role, and stress; and the *social system* is composed of the concepts of organization, decision making, power, authority, and status.

A diagnostic category, according to NANDA, consists of (a) the definition of the diagnosis, (b) the related factors (or the probable cause of the problem), and (c) the defining characteristics (or signs and symptoms). Two methods of categorizing NANDA's nursing diagnoses according to the concepts within King's conceptual framework were attempted by the Nursing Practice Committee.

An initial attempt at using related factors as the basis for linking diagnoses to concepts was abandoned in favor of using defining characteristics. When related factors were used, diagnoses fell into numerous systems and concepts, and this method was deemed unwieldy. A second drawback was that nurses tended to focus on the related factors before clustering defining characteristics, which could possibly lead to a premature incorrect diagnosis.

The second method involved linking a diagnosis based on the associated list of defining characteristics to a concept. The latter system, herein described, was preferred because defining characteristics represent the clinically based empirical data that nurses observe in daily practice that lead them to make clinical judgments.

Methods

The preliminary categorization of the NANDA list of nursing diagnoses according to King's three systems was completed by the Nursing Practice Committee. Members of this committee had spent almost 2 years studying King's conceptual framework and assisting in its implementation and more than a year becoming familiar with the use of nursing diagnoses. Through discussion of definitions of the nursing diagnoses and defining characteristics, each nursing diagnosis was tied to a particular concept within one of three systems in King's conceptual framework. In order to facilitate categorization, King's concept of *growth and development* was subdivided in order to accommodate the nursing diagnoses that deal with specific body systems. This, however, was in keeping with King's definition of that concept (King, 1981, p. 169). To categorize those nursing diagnoses that did not fit into a discrete biologic system, the category of "multiple biological systems" was created.

Following initial categorization, the committee sought to determine whether nurses who had not studied nursing diagnoses as intensively as had committee members could link a nursing diagnosis to one of King's concepts (preferably the same concept chosen by the committee) based on the defining characteristics of the diagnosis. The committee enlisted the help of the Nursing Audit Committee, a 17-member subcommittee that comprised the other half of the Nursing Quality Assurance Committee and represented nurses from all levels. The committee members had knowledge of King's framework, but their knowledge of nursing diagnoses was more general than that of the Nursing Practice Committee.

During the first round of categorization, each nurse was given the task of linking each nursing diagnosis with a concept from King's framework through a pencil and paper exercise that required simple matching. For example, the nursing diagnosis anxiety was linked with King's concept of *perception*. In choosing concepts with the best fit, nurses used their knowledge of the definitions of King's concepts and the definitions and defining characteristics of the diagnostic labels. All of this information was available in written form during the matching. A nursing diagnosis was considered categorized if it was linked with the same concept by at least 70% of the group.

During the second round, the nursing diagnosis-concept links that did not meet the 70% criterion were reconsidered by the same group. For each of these diagnoses, the group reexamined the most frequently chosen of King's concepts. Each concept was rated by individual nurses for degree of fit with the diagnosis, the choices being (a) poor, (b) slight, (c) good, or (d) excellent. A nursing diagnosis was considered categorized if 70% of the group isolated the same concept as having a good or excellent fit.

Results

Thirty-nine of the 83 diagnoses accepted by NANDA after the Seventh National Conference on Classification of Nursing Diagnoses in 1986 were classified by the Nursing Audit Committee after the first round.

Thirty-nine of the 44 diagnoses that had not been considered as categorized in the first round met the criterion in the second round. That is, at least 70% of nurses in the group agreed that a given diagnosis-concept link had a good or excellent fit. Classification of a nursing diagnosis within a single concept was not always possible because in some situations the nursing diagnosis was found to have the same degree of fit with two concepts. In these few cases, the Nursing Practice Committee decided to allow the same diagnosis to appear under two headings in the categorization tool.

Finalization of the categorization tool was completed by a panel of experts that consisted of three directors of nursing, a clinical nurse specialist, a clinical instructor, and a staff nurse. Their decisions were based on the results of the first two rounds of categorization. In the five cases where categorization was not possible based on the stated criterion, the expert panel relied on the results of the preliminary work by the Nursing Practice Committee. This expert panel also updated the tool a year later by fitting new diagnoses into the existing concept categories after the results of the Eighth National NANDA conference were published (Kim, McFarland, & McLane, 1989). The expert panel alone was used to categorize the additional nursing diagnoses primarily for three reasons:

1. The Quality Assurance Committee, which was composed of the Nursing Practice and Audit Subcommittees, was disbanded in favor of a new committee structure and original committee members had assumed positions on the new committees.
2. The diagnoses to be added were straightforward with respect to suitable categorization. Agreement among panel members was well above the 70% standard in all cases at the outset, and consensus was readily achieved.
3. Time was of some concern at this point with respect to completing the implementation process.

The final categorization of nursing diagnoses according to the systems and concepts of King's conceptual framework can be seen in Table 13.1.

Stage 2:
Testing the Utility of the Nursing Diagnoses Categorization Tool

Following finalization of the categorization tool, a study was conducted to determine whether the tool could assist nurses to connect NANDA's nursing diagnoses with King's conceptual framework.

Methods

Nursing managers on three continuing care units and one rehabilitation unit were asked for a list of nurses who had been working on the units for at least 1 year and who worked at least part-time. It was assumed that these nurses were familiar with King's conceptual framework because they had participated in a project over the past 16 months through which they were exposed to the concepts in the framework (Byrne & Schreiber, 1989). The nurses had not, however, been taught specifically about nursing diagnoses. A total of 28 nurses were randomly selected from this list. The first 3 nurses were used in a pilot study to test the feasibility of the study design. No significant changes were made in the protocol as a result.

TABLE 13.1   Categorization of NANDA Nursing Diagnoses According to the Systems and Concepts of King's Conceptual Framework

PERSONAL SYSTEM

Perception
  Anxiety
  Fear
  Grieving, anticipatory
  Grieving, dysfunctional
  Knowledge deficit (specify)
  Pain
  Pain, chronic
  Sensory/perceptual alterations:
    visual, auditory, kinesthetic,
    gustatory, tactile, olfactory
  Social isolation
  Thought processes, altered
  Unilateral neglect
Self and Body Image
  Body image disturbance
  Coping, defensive
  Growth and development, altered
  Hopelessness
  Personal identity disturbance
  Powerlessness
  Self-esteem, chronic low
  Self-esteem, disturbance
  Self-esteem, situational low
  Sexual dysfunction
  Sexuality patterns, altered
  Spiritual distress (distress of the
    human spirit)
  Violence, potential for: self-directed
    or directed at others
Space and Time
  Diversional activity deficit
Growth and Development[a]
  Cardiovascular System
    Activity intolerance
    Activity intolerance: potential
    Cardiac output: decreased
  Respiratory System
    Activity intolerance
    Activity intolerance: potential
    Airway clearance, ineffective
    Aspiration, potential for
    Breathing pattern, ineffective
    Gas exchange, impaired

PERSONAL SYSTEM (Cont'd)

Neurological System
  Dysreflexia
  Sensory/perceptual alterations
    (specify): visual, auditory,
    kinesthetic, gustatory, tactile,
    olfactory
  Sleep pattern disturbance
  Unilateral neglect
Gastrointestinal System
  Bowel incontinence
  Constipation
  Constipation, colonic
  Constipation, perceived
  Diarrhea
  Nutrition, altered: less than body
    requirements
  Nutrition, altered: more than
    body requirements
  Nutrition, altered: potential for
    more than body requirements
  Oral mucous membrane, altered
  Swallowing, impaired
Genitourinary System
  Incontinence, functional
  Incontinence, reflex
  Incontinence, stress
  Incontinence, total
  Incontinence, urge
  Urinary elimination, altered
    patterns
  Urinary retention
Integumentary System
  Skin integrity, impaired
  Skin integrity, impaired potential
Musculoskeletal System
  Disuse syndrome, potential for
  Mobility, impaired physical
  Self-care deficit, bathing/ hygiene
  Self-care deficit, dressing/
    grooming
  Self-care deficit, feeding
  Self-care deficit, toileting
Multiple Biological System
  Body temperature, altered,
    potential

(continued)

TABLE 13.1 Continued

PERSONAL SYSTEM (Cont'd)	INTERPERSONAL SYSTEM (Cont'd)
Fatigue	Coping, ineffective individual
Fluid volume deficit (1)	Denial, ineffective
Fluid volume deficit (2)	Health maintenance, altered
Fluid volume deficit, potential	Infection, potential for
Fluid volume excess	Injury, potential for
Growth and development, altered	Poisoning, potential for
Hyperthermia	Post trauma response
Hypothermia	Rape-trauma syndrome
Thermoregulation, ineffective	Rape-trauma syndrome: compound
Tissue integrity, impaired	reaction
Tissue perfusion, altered: renal,	Rape-trauma syndrome: silent
cerebral, cardiopulmonary,	reaction
gastrointestinal, peripheral	Suffocation, potential for
	Trauma, potential for
INTERPERSONAL SYSTEM	
Interaction	**SOCIAL SYSTEM**
Social interaction, impaired	**Organization**
Communication	Coping, family: potential for growth
Communication, impaired verbal	Coping, ineffective family:
Transaction	compromised
Health-seeking behaviors (specify)	Coping, ineffective family: disabling
Noncompliance (specify)	Family processes, altered
Role	Home maintenance management,
Breast-feeding, ineffective	impaired
Parental role conflict	**Authority, Power**
Parenting, altered: actual/potential	**Status**
Role performance, altered	**Decision making**
Stress	Decisional conflict (specify)
Adjustment, impaired	

a. Systems in this category constitute a modification of King's framework by the Nursing Practice Committee based on King's patient database (King, 1981, p. 109).

Each of the remaining 25 nurses was approached individually and, after the study design was explained, was asked to participate. Two who chose not to participate were replaced with two randomly selected nurses.

Each participant was asked to complete an exercise (see Figure 13.1) to determine the thought processes used to organize relevant data in selecting a nursing diagnosis. In this exercise, the nurse was given the defining characteristics of a nursing diagnosis and was asked to describe on paper the steps used to arrive at a diagnosis. Subjects were allowed to use any resource material they were in the habit of

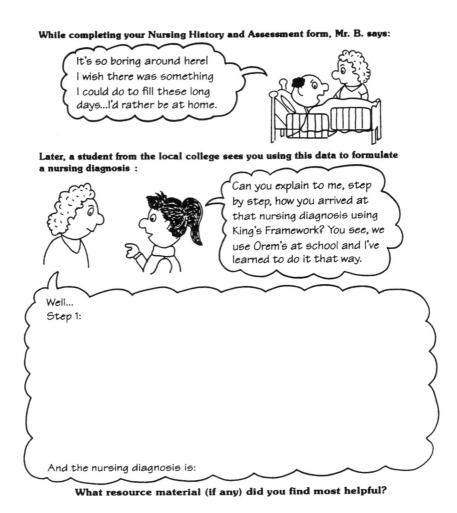

Figure 13.1. Exercise for Recording Nurses' Thought Processes as They Formulate a Nursing Diagnosis

using. Each completed exercise sheet was coded with a symbol known only to the subject. Upon completion of the exercise, the nurse was given a self-directed learning package on care planning and nursing diagnoses that took 1 hour to complete. This package provided some background on the use of nursing diagnoses; explained how to cluster cues in order to arrive at a diagnosis; and described how to write a diagnosis, expected outcomes, and nursing interventions and to evaluate nursing care.

One week later, each nurse attended an in-service educational session with two or three other participants. At the 40-minute session, questions regarding nursing diagnoses were answered and nurses received a copy of the categorization tool. Use of the tool was explained, and subjects had time to practice arriving at a nursing diagnosis after receiving some defining characteristics.

Nurse subjects were asked to practice writing nursing diagnoses on their care plans and to use the new tool as a reference. Over the next 4 weeks they practiced using the tool. Those who found it easier to use case studies rather than their own patients were given the opportunity to do so. A clinical instructor was available during this time to check care plans and to help nurses arrive at a diagnosis if necessary. The clinical instructor checked in with each nurse on a few occasions throughout the trial period to ensure that the nurse was able to use the tool.

Approximately 4 weeks later, each nurse repeated the same exercise. Subjects were again asked which resource material was most helpful. Answer sheets were coded as before. The two exercises were matched by the symbols, and the responses in both exercises were compared.

Results

A panel consisting of a director of nursing, a clinical nurse specialist, a clinical instructor, and a staff nurse analyzed the content of the completed exercises. They completed score sheets for each pair of exercises, noting the presence or absence of certain criteria used to indicate whether a connection had been made between the formulation of the nursing diagnosis and King's conceptual framework throughout the nurse's thought processes. The panel of experts outlined these criteria after they had reviewed the literature on the process of nursing diagnosis. The panel agreed that the early part of the diagnostic process consists of clustering cues and applying a diagnostic label based on the defining characteristics of a nursing

TABLE 13.2   Percentage of Nurses Meeting the Criteria for Making a Connection With King's Framework While Formulating a Nursing Diagnosis (*N* = 25)

Criteria	Pretest (%)	Posttest (%)
Reference to King's conceptual framework	8	32
Reference to the fact that one of King's systems should be considered	16	80
Choice of the correct system (i.e., personal system)	4	60
Reference to the fact that one of King's concepts should be considered	8	72
Choice of the correct concept (i.e., time)	0	44
Comparison of collected data with the defining characteristics associated with the NANDA diagnosis	4	44
Choice of the correct nursing diagnosis (i.e., diversional activity deficit)	12	44
Identification of the nursing diagnoses categorization tool as the most useful reference	—	52[a]

a. 32% (*n* = 8) of nurses failed to respond to this question.

diagnosis. The panel also wished to determine whether the nurse could recognize which of King's concepts was associated with the cues gathered. The criteria used to determine the nurse's thought processes evolved through integration of these steps. The criteria and the percentage of participants meeting the criteria during the pretest and posttest are shown in Table 13.2.

The McNemar test for the significance of changes (Siegel, 1956) showed that in the posttest, the nurses showed a significant tendency to

1. Make reference to King's conceptual framework ($\chi^2 = 3.125, p < .05$)
2. Make more specific reference to one of King's systems ($\chi^2 = 14.45$, $p < .0005$)
3. Make more specific reference to one of King's concepts ($\chi^2 = 13.47$, $p < .0005$)
4. Match collected data with the defining characteristics associated with a NANDA diagnosis ($\chi^2 = 6.75, p < .005$)
5. Change from an incorrect diagnostic label to a correct label ($\chi^2 = 7.1$, $p < .005$)

6. Change reference materials in favor of the nursing diagnoses categorization tool ($\chi^2 = 6.125, p < .01$)

Discussion

A tool that categorizes NANDA nursing diagnoses according to the systems and concepts of King's conceptual framework was designed by nurses who were in the process of implementing King's framework to guide practice in the nursing department. The goal was to develop a tool that would assist nurses to make accurate nursing diagnoses following data gathering guided by the conceptual framework.

Tool Development

Categorization of NANDA's nursing diagnoses into King's systems was accomplished through a process involving a large group of nurses experienced with King's conceptual framework. The advantage of involving a large group of people in the categorization process, rather than relying solely on a panel of experts, was that the group as a whole felt committed to the finished product. An expert panel completed the process of categorizing the small number of diagnoses that remained unclassified after two rounds of categorization by the large group.

The relatively small sample size and use of a convenience sample resulted in decreased external validity of the categorization tool. The knowledge of King's conceptual framework and nursing diagnoses possessed by members of the Nursing Audit Committee who participated in the two rounds of categorization was not directly assessed. It may not have been at the expected level, which was assumed to be closer to that of the Nursing Practice Committee members than that of a typical staff nurse. This may have accounted for only 39 diagnoses being satisfactorily categorized during the first round. There may have been some merit, however, in the knowledge levels closely approximating those of staff nurses since the tool would eventually be used by staff nurses.

Tool Implementation

After being introduced to the tool, 80% of nurses made reference to the fact that one of King's systems should be considered when formulating a NANDA nursing diagnosis. Seventy-two percent of the nurses made reference to the fact that one of King's concepts should be considered. The choice of the correct system, concept, and diagnosis was not always accurate, but there was a significant increase in accuracy in the posttest. Twenty-three nurses (92%) improved the overall accuracy of their answers in the posttest.

The improvement in the degree of accuracy found on the posttest may have been related to a factor other than the use of the categorization tool alone. Use of the self-directed learning package and the small-group instruction may have influenced the results. Since the Department of Nursing wanted to introduce nursing diagnoses in relation to King's framework, it was not feasible to teach nursing diagnosis without the tool, and the tool alone was useless without prior knowledge of the diagnostic process.

Although nurses verbally endorsed the categorization tool, it was difficult to conclude whether they felt that the tool was a better reference for arriving at nursing diagnoses than the pocket guides to nursing diagnoses available on their units. Only 52% of respondents indicated that the categorization tool was their most useful reference; 32% of the subjects did not answer the question. This may have been related to the somewhat inconspicuous placement of the item on the exercise sheet, although this was not a problem apparent during the pilot test.

Implications and Summary

Implementation of a nursing conceptual framework is a difficult process requiring constant reinforcement in order for the framework to be internalized by the nurses working within it. It becomes necessary to tie as many activities as possible into the implementation process so that use of a conceptual framework is not seen as an activity far removed from everyday nursing practice. A variation of the process used in this article could be used by groups of nurses regardless of the conceptual framework they have chosen.

Categorizing nursing diagnoses according to the concepts in a nursing framework and providing this resource for nurses may make the framework more meaningful. It also may decrease the confusion caused by introducing nurses to a classification method that does not seem consistent with the framework that guides their practice.

The process of developing and testing the categorization tool produced a core group of nurses from all levels who grew in their knowledge of King's conceptual framework and nursing diagnoses through analysis and critical appraisal of the validity of concept-diagnosis links. Others with whom they worked became curious about the categorization tool and the project itself, and the participants found themselves explaining the connection between nursing diagnoses and King's framework to their colleagues. Other areas of the hospital eagerly awaited completion of the project so the tool could be used as a teaching aid.

The purpose of designing the categorization tool was to assist nurses to identify more clearly the connection between a theoretical base and the formulation of NANDA nursing diagnoses. The results indicated that nurses were better able to make a connection between NANDA's nursing diagnoses and King's conceptual framework with the assistance of a nursing diagnoses categorization tool and some in-service instruction.

The dynamic nature of nursing diagnostic definitions and defining characteristics and the conceptual framework results in any attempt at categorization being tentative at best. It is acknowledged that input from practicing nurses and the incorporation of changes made at future NANDA conferences will necessitate ongoing revisions of this categorization tool.

References

Byrne, E., & Schreiber, R. (1989). Concept of the month; Implementing King's conceptual framework at the bedside. *Journal of Nursing Administration, 19*(2), 28-32.

Kim, M., McFarland, G., & McLane, A. (1989). *Pocket guide to nursing diagnoses* (3rd ed.). St. Louis, MO: C. V. Mosby.

King, I. (1981). *A theory for nursing: Systems, concepts, process.* New York: John Wiley.

Martin, P., & Frank, B. (1989). NANDA nursing diagnostic categories and their relationship to specific nursing theories. In R. M. Carroll-Johnson (Ed.), *Classification of nursing diagnoses: Proceedings of the eighth conference* (pp. 411-413). Philadelphia: J. B. Lippincott.

Siegel, S. (1956). *Nonparametric statistics for the behavioral sciences.* New York: McGraw-Hill.

— 14 —

Integration of King's Framework Into Nursing Practice

J. MARY FAWCETT

VALINE M. VAILLANCOURT

C. ANNABELLE WATSON

Is patient care enhanced by the adoption of a conceptual framework?

Can nurses apply the concepts and tenets of a framework at the bedside?

Can this be done without conflict with individual nurses' own theoretical approaches?

These questions, initially asked within the Departments of Nursing at the Hamilton Civic Hospitals in the mid-1980s, laid the groundwork for many changes in nursing practice. The process of selecting an appropriate conceptual framework, planning for change, implementing new practices, and evaluating the results is discussed in this chapter. Principles of planned change, organizational support, teaching and learning, and shared involvement were as essential to the implementation process as the incorporation of the framework concepts into the philosophy, standards, and nursing process.

Selection of King's Conceptual Framework

The Hamilton Civic Hospitals, a large tertiary care facility in southwestern Ontario, is composed of two geographically separate divisions, each with a Department of Nursing. In October 1985, the nursing executives of both divisions began meeting in response to a statement from the College of Nurses of Ontario (1985). The College of Nurses, in defining their assumptive base for the new provincial standards of nursing practice, said that the practice of nursing was changing from an activity-oriented vocation to a goal-directed profession and that it was essential to put increased emphasis on nursing knowledge and nursing theories.

The nursing executives wanted to examine the feasibility of adopting a common conceptual framework that would reflect the proposed new provincial standards of nursing practice. The project of implementing a conceptual framework for nursing practice was to be the first joint effort of both Departments of Nursing. A nursing practice coordinator was appointed to plan and coordinate the project; however, it soon became apparent that a broader administrative decision-making group was needed for communication and accountability. This support was seen as crucial to the success of implementation. Thus the Nursing Council, consisting of senior nursing executives, was formed.

The first task of this group was the selection of a framework. Following a series of presentations about the works of various theorists, all nurse managers and nurse clinicians were involved in the final selection of one theorist. King's (1981) conceptual framework was chosen for several reasons: (a) It was based on a systems approach, which was thought to offer flexibility in caring for patients in all settings of the hospitals; (b) it viewed the patient in a holistic manner, which would allow nurses to consider all phases of treatment, including psychosocial considerations and discharge planning;

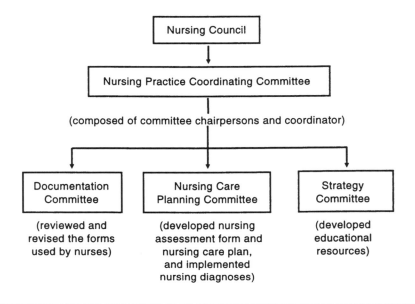

Figure 14.1.   Committee Structure for Implementation of the King Project

and (c) it included the interaction between the nurse and the patient with an emphasis on patient goals. It was hoped that this framework would support a change in both perception and practice from nurses doing things *to* patients to nurses doing things *with* patients and their families.

Operational Structure
for Implementation

Once King's conceptual framework (1981) was selected by the Departments of Nursing, a committee structure was developed to plan and coordinate the implementation process. The Nursing Practice Coordinating Committee was directly responsible for the Nursing Council and for three subcommittees: Nursing Care Planning, Documentation, and Strategy (see Figure 14.1). There were nursing representatives from each division on these committees.

It was important that these representatives included all levels of staff. Nurse managers were necessary in relation to considering both budget and performance expectations, whereas nurse clinicians offered skills in the development of educational plans and resources. In addition, staff nurses were critical to the planning process if King's conceptual framework was to be used effectively at the patient's bedside.

Nursing Practice Coordinating Committee

The purpose of the Nursing Practice Coordinating Committee was to facilitate consistency of nursing practice within the Departments of Nursing using King's conceptual framework. This committee was made up of a nursing executive from each division and the chairpersons of the three subcommittees. Their first step was to ensure that the philosophy of the nursing departments reflected this framework. Because the values and beliefs of these departments were already consistent with the four central concepts of the metaparadigm of nursing (individual, health, nursing, and environment), it was only necessary to edit the philosophy (see the appendix) to incorporate the terminology used in King's framework.

Once the philosophy was revised, the Nursing Practice Coordinating Committee then proceeded to integrate the framework with the standards of nursing practice for the departments. These standards were concurrently under review to meet the revised standards of nursing practice established by the College of Nurses of Ontario (1990). The departments' standards of nursing practice identified expectations for registered nurses and registered practical nurses in providing patient care and were used as a basis for performance appraisal. Performance appraisal criteria for registered nurses and registered practical nurses were then revised to reflect the new standards.

After revising the philosophy and standards of nursing practice to reflect King's conceptual framework, the role of this committee involved the following:

1. Identifying and operationalizing the changes that were necessary to reflect the use of the conceptual framework in the delivery of patient care

2. Acting as a steering committee for the development of an implementation plan with time lines
3. Coordinating and approving the activities of the subcommittees
4. Reporting the progress of implementation to the Nursing Council
5. Discussing budgetary implications with the Nursing Council
6. Evaluating the progress and effectiveness of implementation

Nursing Care Planning Committee

The Nursing Care Planning Committee was responsible for developing a system for implementation of the nursing process using King's conceptual framework. Their initial objective was to review and revise the admission nursing assessment form. This review resulted in the development of an assessment form that used the concepts from King as the headings to categorize information. The form was divided into three sections to reflect King's three systems: personal, interpersonal, and social. The form was also divided vertically to facilitate documentation of both the patient's perceptions and the nurse's perceptions. The questions were worded to facilitate ease of comprehension so that patients, when possible, could complete the patient's perception side of the form.

Concurrent with the adoption of King's conceptual framework, the Departments of Nursing decided to implement the use of nursing diagnoses in care planning. The North American Nursing Diagnosis Association (NANDA) diagnostic statements (Kim, McFarland, & McLane, 1989) were used to give direction to nursing staff. The NANDA diagnoses (Kim et al., 1989) were divided into King's 15 concepts. Byrne-Coker et al. (1990) used a similar method of categorization in their implementation process. The basic premise was that repeated use of the diagnostic list, categorized under the conceptual framework, would reinforce the nurses' exposure to King's concepts.

To further reinforce the use of King's conceptual framework, the nursing care plan was revised to include columns for nursing diagnosis, patient goals, nursing actions, and evaluation. In the goals column, statements were to be identified as either nursing or mutual. In actuality, this strengthened the concepts of King's goal attainment, care planning, and nursing diagnoses.

Documentation Committee

The Documentation Committee was to develop a documentation package that supported King's conceptual framework and the philosophy of the Departments of Nursing. Documentation must be done by all nurses, regardless of their work setting or role. Because documentation is a daily practice familiar to nurses, the decision was made to link the conceptual framework to charting.

The nurses' notes posed a particular challenge. The Documentation Committee was faced with the question of how the major concepts and themes of King's framework could be incorporated into a realistic documentation system. Following a review of the literature on problem-oriented charting and focus charting (Iyer & Camp, 1991), it was decided to combine these two approaches.

In relation to problem-oriented charting, the emphasis was placed on a goal orientation rather than on a problem orientation. This change in orientation reflected King's concepts and reinforced the need for mutual goal setting between the patient and nurse. This led to the development of SOGIE charting (Vaillancourt, 1994). The acronym SOGIE stands for subjective, objective, goal, implementation of nursing actions, and evaluation. SOGIE charting provides nurses with a mechanism for identifying and reviewing patient goals on a daily or regular basis.

Focus charting was incorporated into documentation on the nurses' notes through the use of notations. If the nurse was not charting a nursing diagnosis, the word *notation* could be written in the nursing diagnosis/notation column and the information charted to its right. Nurses used the notation approach to document assessment or incidents that did not pertain to the care plan or that were unusual or single occurrences. Many nurses found that they preferred to use the SOGIE format even when documenting a notation because it provides a consistent framework for thinking and writing.

To facilitate the move away from narrative charting of the patient's basic care activities, a personal systems flow sheet was developed. Space was provided on this form for the identification of individual patient care needs. This form allowed nurses to initial the routine aspects of daily care and to indicate with a circled *NN* if there was an additional reference on the nurses' notes.

Concurrent with these documentation changes, a patient assessment/teaching flow sheet was introduced. This form included educational goals, teaching strategies, evaluation of goal attainment, and discharge educational needs and was developed for specific diseases or treatments (Hilts, 1991).

These changes in documentation were relevant only to those patient care areas that used care plans and nurses' notes. There were several areas, such as the Post-Anesthetic Recovery Room, critical care units, Operating Room, Emergency Department, and Ambulatory Care Department, that had replaced the traditional forms with flow sheets and unit-specific documentation forms. The Documentation Committee worked with these areas to assist them in adapting their own forms to both nursing diagnoses and King's concepts.

Strategy Committee

The Strategy Committee, the third subcommittee of the Nursing Practice Coordinating Committee, was responsible for planning and coordinating the education and information strategies for the introduction of King's conceptual framework and the expected changes in nursing practice. Because King described people as rational and purposeful in their behavior, this committee felt that the implementation of King's framework in both divisions must also be rational and purposeful. If change was going to occur and be effective, it was important that the staff nurse at the bedside experience a sense of meaning and practicality relatively early in the change process (Fullan, 1982).

During the planning and development stage, a series of bulletins briefly outlining King's basic concepts were sent to all of the clinical areas. These were posted on purple backdrops and updated on a monthly basis. A conceptual framework logo was designed that used vectors to represent the problem-solving or decision-making processes. These vectors terminated in various directions but emanated primarily from within a loosely defined cubic scaffold or framework forming the letter K. This logo was used repeatedly throughout the development and implementation process (Homerski, 1987).

A video was produced that demonstrated the use of King's conceptual framework in nursing practice. A self-directed workbook was developed and distributed to each nurse to assist in the application of relevant concepts to the patient. Both the video and workbook were used in the education process. Overheads and slides were also produced to assist with implementation and to provide consistency in the delivery of in-services. In addition, case studies were developed that demonstrated the application of King's concepts to practice within a variety of patient situations.

Seven days prior to the actual implementation of King's framework on a unit, the Kountdown Kalendar was posted to generate enthusiasm among nursing staff. The nurse clinician on the unit was responsible for tearing off the top page until "K-Day" arrived. To support the use of the concepts once King's framework had been implemented on a unit, Koncept of the Month was introduced. Based on work by Byrne and Schreiber (1989), each of the 15 concepts was printed on a separate page with a definition and two questions regarding its application to the patient and the nurse, respectively. These were to be posted on the purple backdrops and used to generate discussion among staff nurses. The ordering of the concepts would be decided by the nurse clinician depending on the needs of the patients and staff.

Implementation

Implementation of King's conceptual framework throughout the Departments of Nursing required the support of the nurse clinicians, nurse managers, and nursing administration.

The nurse manager's role was to act as the key person responsible for the coordination and implementation of King's framework on their nursing unit. The nurse clinicians were the key resource persons for the teaching, integration, and implementation of King's conceptual framework and for nursing care planning.

In addition, nursing staff from each of the clinical areas were identified as "King preceptors" to assist in the implementation process. These preceptors acted as a resource for their peers in relation to King's framework and its application through assessment, care planning, and documentation. They also worked with the nurse manager and clinician to individualize King's framework to the needs of their clinical area.

All nurse managers, nurse clinicians, and King preceptors received a 7-hour educational session on King's conceptual framework, its application to practice, the implementation process, and resources available. All nursing staff received 4 hours of educational classes delivered by a unit-based clinician.

All units were involved in the implementation process. However, to allow for a review of both the process and the educational resources, the project was phased in over 24 months. The initial pilot on one medical and one surgical unit at each division continued for approximately 6 months. A pre- and postimplementation audit of documentation on these units was completed for comparison and evaluation purposes.

Implementation throughout the remaining units involved five phases over an 18-month period. During each phase, two or three units at each division were introduced to the conceptual framework and documentation forms. Unit clinicians assisted one another with the delivery of classes to the staff.

Through the use of the documentation system, the nursing staff became familiar with the language of King. The familiarity with the language and visualization of the concepts led the staff of an active surgical unit to appreciate the need to use King's conceptual framework, as demonstrated in the following example.

Case Application

The nursing staff on an acute care surgical unit had an experience with a patient that gave them an awareness of how King's conceptual framework could guide their nursing practice (Arnold, Eddy, Forler, & Rawlin, 1991).

The patient, K. C., was a 41-year-old married mother of four school-age children. A university graduate, she had worked outside the home for several years. K. C. had been relatively healthy with no major illnesses until she discovered a marble-sized lump in her left breast. A left partial mastectomy with axillary node dissection was performed. Four of six nodes were positive for malignant disease, but a bone scan was negative for metastaic disease.

Four weeks after surgery, K. C. started chemotherapy treatments that continued over the next 6 months. Throughout this period, both she and her husband were very anxious about her diagnosis and prognosis. She experienced nausea, vomiting, and diarrhea. Both the treatments and the symptoms continued throughout the summer months, and she came to dread the sessions more and more. In August, after the fifth of seven treatments, she was admitted to the hospital with fever, neutropenia, diarrhea, and rectal bleeding. It was determined that the lower portion of her bowel was inflamed and ulcerated and chemotherapy was discontinued. She was discharged home in early October.

Within 3 weeks, K. C. returned through the Emergency Department with severe left abdominal pain, watery diarrhea, and abdominal distention. She was admitted with toxic megacolon to the intensive care unit (ICU), where she was rehydrated, transfused, administered antibiotics and analgesics, and observed carefully over the next few days. Following perforation of both her large and small bowel, she had a subtotal colectomy with formation of ileostomy and mucous fistula.

Postoperatively, she did not do well and eventually required a permanent ileostomy. It was a difficult time for K. C. and her family. She was septic, immunocompromised, ventilated, and often delirious. It was in fact a time of depression and despair. After 2 weeks the sepsis started to abate and her condition began to improve sufficiently for her to be moved out of the ICU.

It was at this time that K. C. arrived on the active surgical unit. She expressed no desire to do anything and preferred to spend the day just lying on her bed. She often asked the nurses to leave her alone, proclaiming that she couldn't do the task requested. Because this was just 5 to 6 weeks before Christmas, everyone assumed that K. C. wanted to be home for Christmas. Nurses, doctors, and even family were making goals for K. C. and trying to reassure her that it would be fun to go home. Although K. C. continued to state that she was not going, Christmas finally arrived and K. C. did go home for a 24-hour period.

She returned more withdrawn and more helpless than before. The nurses frequently held conferences to talk about a possible plan for her. Other disciplines were involved on a regular basis, and hours were spent trying to talk with her to discover the source of the problem. K. C. barely responded to these efforts and showed very little emotion even to her family. She refused to look at her ileostomy or have anything to do with it. The nurses became increasingly frustrated with K. C.'s lack of progress and the time involved in her care. It took 30 to 45 minutes to get her from a supine position to a standing position at the bedside.

It was at this time that the nurses were introduced to King's conceptual framework. Aware of the need for patient involvement in goal setting, they hoped to come up with one goal that would help her to turn around. As a short-term measure, they revised their plan for daily care activities with some direction from K. C. New goals were set and written on poster board so that they could be hung on her walls for her to see. Basically, they included a progression in mobility from "raise head of bed" to "walk in room." Despite these posted goals, K. C. continued to refuse to participate, complaining that she was in too much pain. Her constant cry was "Leave me alone, please!"

The nurses realized that their goal chart was not the answer to patient involvement and control. They felt increasingly helpless. It seemed that the more they tried, the less response they got. Throughout this period K. C.'s depression became more pronounced as she experienced continuing medical problems that required long-term antibiotics, parenteral nutrition, frequent catheterizations, and repeat wound dressings. Despite all of the problems, the order to mobilize was maintained because there was no physical evidence of a disease condition preventing such.

Recognizing that K. C. might relate better to a few select nurses who wanted to work with her and that she would benefit from continuity of care, the ward assignment was changed to facilitate a group of consistent nurses. Approximately 3 months after Christmas, K. C. was diagnosed with osteomyelitis of the spine. Both the nurses and K. C. now had a reason for her pain; the nurses could understand her protests, and K. C. could regain her self-esteem because her problems were not perceived as psychological. She was placed on bed rest for several weeks on a special bed designed to decrease risk of skin breakdown. The change was remarkable. K. C. started to smile and talk more, even laugh.

During this period, the nurses discovered in talking with K. C. that she was an avid fan of a popular Canadian female vocalist. She revealed that she and her husband had tickets to a special concert by this performer that included a wine and cheese party afterward and that she very much wanted to go. This became the goal for both K. C. and the nurses, one that was indeed mutually identified. In looking back at this experience, the nurses realized that K. C. had set her own goal and that it had nothing to do with mobility, self-care, resuming the role of wife/mother/daughter, or even being a model patient. It had to do with her love of music and was as simple as the hoped-for attendance at a special concert.

Both K. C. and the nurses realized that if they were going to achieve this goal, K. C. needed to be as independent as possible. This was aided by the move to a different bed that still provided protection from skin breakdown but permitted K. C. to operate it herself. From this point on, the advances were clearly noticeable. K. C. progressed to a walker and was able to go on outings with her family. She did attend the special concert and met the performer in person, thus accomplishing her identified goal. She was eventually transferred to the rehabilitation floor for continuing therapy and was finally discharged from the hospital, walking with two canes.

In summary, the nursing staff of this surgical unit had worked with K. C. over a 14-month period, dealing with continuing physiological, psychosocial, and spiritual needs. They experienced frustration and uncertainty when they tried to coordinate her care, because K. C.'s perceptions and goals were not congruent with their perceptions and goals for her care. With the introduction of King's conceptual framework, the nurses became more aware of both K. C.'s and their own personal systems and sought to involve her totally in goal setting. It was not, however, until the goal became truly mutual that the nurses and K. C. were able to progress together toward goal achievement and a state of health for K. C. that allowed her to achieve her maximum potential for daily living.

Through this experience, the nurses on this surgical unit were able to gain both an awareness and an appreciation of how King's conceptual framework can guide nursing practice to enhance quality patient care. For these nurses, this was an excellent preface to the introduction of theory-based practice at the Hamilton Civic Hospitals.

Ongoing Work

The nurses at the Hamilton Civic Hospitals continue to provide nursing care based on King's conceptual framework. The Nursing Council Committee and the Nursing Practice Coordinating Committee have proved to be such an effective method of coordinating projects within the Departments of Nursing that they continue to meet on a regular basis. Because these committees no longer need to focus their attention on the implementation of a conceptual framework, they now coordinate practice within the Departments of Nursing. Both the Nursing Care Planning and Strategy Committees have completed their tasks and have dissolved. The Documentation Committee has evolved into coordinating the review, revision, and evaluation of all forms within the Departments of Nursing.

The Standards of Patient Care Committee has been initiated to automate the nursing care planning system. This committee has developed standards of patient care using diagnoses from NANDA (Kim et al., 1989). Standards of patient care have been developed for individual diagnoses as well as for diagnoses grouped according to condition or disease. For example, a standard of patient care has been developed for the diagnosis of acute pain and another standard of patient care has been developed for a grouping of diagnoses titled "pre-operative care."

Specific measurable patient goals have been identified for each diagnosis and are labeled as either "nursing" or "mutual." These goals will be used to measure the effectiveness of care.

The quality assurance program reflects concepts from King's conceptual framework but to date does not measure the outcomes of the care given. It is anticipated that the goals identified in the standards of patient care will be used to determine outcomes and the effectiveness of nursing actions.

Summary

Over a 7-year period, the Departments of Nursing have worked collaboratively to provide quality patient care through the implementation of a conceptual framework. King's (1981) conceptual framework has assisted in the review and organization of the philosophy, standards, and nursing process.

King's conceptual framework is now a thread that weaves through all aspects of the Departments of Nursing. For example, a preceptor program has recently been developed on the basis of King's framework, including a learning plan in which a preceptee and preceptor identify their mutual goals and the means of achieving those goals.

As with all change, the adoption and implementation of a conceptual framework is not an event but a process—a process that must permeate all aspects of the delivery of patient care.

Appendix
Hamilton Civic Hospitals
Departments of Nursing

The Departments of Nursing of Hamilton General Division and Henderson General Division, in cooperation with each other, support and facilitate the care of patients along with the educational and research endeavors of these hospitals. We endorse the mission statement of Hamilton Civic Hospitals.

Consistency of nursing practice within the nursing organization is enhanced by the use of a conceptual framework that incorporates beliefs about *the individual, the environment, health,* and *nursing.*

WE BELIEVE THAT

- The *individual* is a unique being with inherent rights and complex needs that are influenced by a number of interacting components. The beliefs, values, and spiritual attributes along with a particular combination of life experiences determine the individual's perception of himself or herself in any one situation.

- The *environment* encompasses both internal and external factors that are physical, psychological, and social in nature. The interaction of these environmental factors influences the individual's relationships, well-being, and behavior.

- *Health* is a dynamic state of optimal functioning. Health requires constant adjustment to stressors in the environment. Altered health states involve imbalances in biological, psychological, and social factors. Individuals perceive their health uniquely and are responsible for its maintenance.

- *Nursing* is composed of practice, research, education, and management. Nursing practice is based on theory, knowledge, and scientific principles. Nurses participate in mutual goal setting with individuals, families, and groups in health promotion and health maintenance. They assist in restoration of optimal health when individuals are unable to do this for themselves. When life cannot be maintained, nurses provide an environment conducive to a peaceful, dignified death. The interdependent functions of nursing are fulfilled in partnership with other members of the health care team.

- *Nursing research* is essential to the ongoing development of nursing practice.

- Our facilitation and contribution to the *education* of nurses and other professionals is essential for the evolution of health care.

- The maintenance of professional competency is the responsibility of each nurse.

- *Management* coordinates and facilitates the achievement of all components of nursing.

References

Arnold, M., Eddy, K., Forler, Y., & Rawlin, D. (1991, February). *Case study: K. C.* Case study presented at Nursing Grand Rounds at the Henderson General Division of the Hamilton Civic Hospitals, Hamilton, Ontario.

Byrne, E., & Schreiber, R. (1989). Concept of the month: Implementing King's conceptual framework at the bedside. *Journal of Nursing Administration, 19*(2), 28-32.

Byrne-Coker, E., Fradley, T., Harris, J., Tomarchio, D., Chan, V., & Caron, C. (1990). Implementing nursing diagnoses within the context of King's conceptual framework. *Nursing Diagnosis, 1*(3), 107-114.

College of Nurses of Ontario. (1985). *Assumptive base for standards of nursing practice.* Toronto, Ontario: Author.

College of Nurses of Ontario. (1990). *Standards of nursing practice for registered nurses and registered nursing assistants.* Toronto, Ontario: Author.

Fullan, M. (1982). *The meaning of educational change.* Toronto: Ontario Institute for Studies in Education.

Hilts, L. (1991). *Patient teaching/assessment flowsheets.* Unpublished manuscript.

Homerski, P. (1987). *Conceptual framework logo.* Unpublished manuscript.

Iyer, P. W., & Camp, N. H. (1991). *Nursing documentation: A nursing process approach.* Toronto, Ontario: C. V. Mosby Year Book.

Kim, M., McFarland, G., & McLane, A. (1989). *A pocket guide to nursing diagnosis.* St. Louis, MO: C. V. Mosby.

King, I. M. (1981). *A theory for nursing: Systems, concepts, process.* New York: John Wiley.

Vaillancourt, V. M. (1994). *Improving the Use of the Nursing Process: The Impact of a Charting Methodology Developed From King's Conceptual Framework on the Use of the Nursing Process.* Unpublished master's thesis, Brock University, St. Catherines, Ontario.

— 15 —

Using King's Systems Framework to Explore Family Health in the Families of the Young Chronically Mentally Ill

MARY MOLEWYK DOORNBOS

It has been estimated that there are approximately 2.5 million chronically mentally ill persons in the United States (Krauss, 1989). Within that number, it appears as though a new chronic psychiatric population is emerging. This population consists of young adults between the ages of 18 and 35 who are seriously impaired in their ability to function socially and psychologically by illnesses such as schizophrenia and bipolar disorders (Wilk, 1988). These young adults do not present as chronically mentally ill in the typical sense because they have only periodic and infrequent contact with the mental health system and, in contrast with older psychiatric clients, have spent little time in the hospital. Their mental illness is, however, clearly of a chronic nature in that it results in significant functional disability.

This new generation of psychiatric clients has been indirectly affected by the deinstitutionalization movement that began in the 1960s. This movement was designed to provide more humane and less restrictive care for the mentally ill by shifting the focus of care from large state mental hospitals to community sites (Kane, 1984). Deinstitutionalization was grounded in the belief that, all things being equal, people fare better in the community than in a restrictive institutional setting. Regrettably, all things have not been equal, and the fundamental support services and resources that were provided by the institution, such as food, clothing, and shelter, have not always been available to the chronically mentally ill in their home communities (Chafetz & Barnes, 1989). In addition, the community treatment alternatives have failed to keep pace with the growing needs of the chronically mentally ill. Thus these young chronic clients, unable to meet their basic needs or obtain adequate services, are dependent on their families for care.

Clearly, then, the impact of a chronic mental illness is not limited to the affected individual. The family of the affected person may be called on to play a major role in the care of their ill member. Lefley (1987) charges that many families took on this awesome caregiving role "not in lieu of, but in lack of, acceptable community alternatives" (p. 1064).

A greater understanding of the experiences and perspective of families caring for a young chronically mentally ill member is necessary. Such an investigation is appropriately undertaken by the discipline of nursing. Nursing seeks to address itself to the human responses of both clients and their families, to actual or potential health problems (American Nurses Association, 1980). Individuals may be responding to their own actual or potential health problems, and families may be responding to the health problems of one of their members. Such a focus recognizes the interaction and interdependence of members of a family unit. Illness in one family member will inevitably affect the rest of the family. In turn, the family unit has the potential for an altered level of health as a result of the difficulties associated with an illness of one of its members. Therefore, nursing's disciplinary focus provides a good fit with a study of the families of the young chronically mentally ill.

The majority of the literature to date pertaining to families with a chronically mentally ill member has used family burden as the entity of interest. There are no studies within this body of literature that explore family health as the outcome variable. Thus there appears to be a need to study this issue from the unique perspective of the discipline of nursing.

King's Systems Framework and Family Health in the Families of the Young Chronically Mentally Ill

King (1968, 1971, 1981, 1990, 1992) has developed and refined a systems framework for nursing that provides the structure for an investigation of the families of the young chronically mentally ill. King makes several basic assumptions about persons, health, environment, and nursing and thus addresses the metaparadigm of the discipline of nursing (Fawcett, 1984). King's development of the metaparadigm concept of person is the most complete. The human being is seen as a unique total system that is open and interacting freely with the environment. The person is further described in terms of three dynamic and interacting systems—personal, interpersonal, and social systems. These systems refer to the individual, groups, and society, respectively, and each is described in terms of relevant concepts (King, 1981, 1992).

Although King's focus was on individuals as the framework was developed, the family has consistently been identified as an important and appropriate system for nurses to address. The family is identified as a basic structural and functional unit of society that engages in the transmission of culture and socialization (King, 1981). King (1981, 1983) has referred to the family as both a social system and an interpersonal system. Furthermore, in stressing the open-systems nature of her framework, King (1992) allows for concepts from each of the systems to be used interchangeably. Thus concepts from the personal, interpersonal, and social systems might be applicable to the family.

King's framework provides the basis for the development of a middle-range theory of family health in the families of the young chronically mentally ill. This middle-range theory development effort conceptualizes the family as an interpersonal system but concepts are used from both personal and interpersonal systems. The middle-range theory explores the relationships between family stressors, family coping, family perception of the client's level of health, time since diagnosis, and the outcome variable of family health. The specific aim of the study was to determine whether or not these factors predicted as well as influenced family health. Each of these concepts had its origin in King's systems framework as well as in the literature pertaining to the families of the chronically mentally ill. The relationships between these variables can be summarized by the diagram in Figure 15.1.

Methods

Design

A predictive, correlational, theory-testing, survey design was used.

Sample

Eighty-four families were obtained by means of a nonprobability sampling strategy. Families were sought from a community mental health agency, public and private psychiatric hospitals, and support groups. The inclusion criteria were as follows: (a) the family must have a young chronically mentally ill member; (b) the family informant(s) must be able to read, write, and speak English; and (c) the young chronically mentally ill member must be characterized by a diagnosis of schizophrenia or bipolar disorder and must be between 18 and 40 years old.

The sample families were predominantly single respondent families from the western Michigan area who were obtained from clinical agencies. On the basis of reported income, the majority of the families were middle-class. Most of the family respondents were white, female, married, college educated parents of the identified client. The

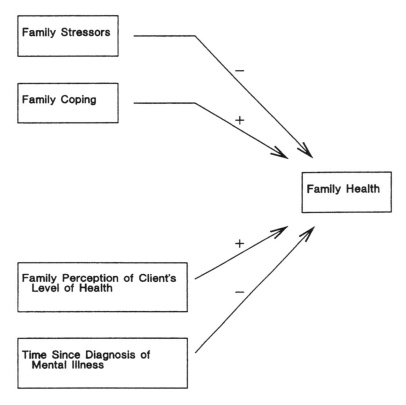

Figure 15.1. Model of the Middle-Range Theory of Family Health in the Families of the Young Chronically Mentally Ill

majority of the clients within these family units were male, had a mean age of approximately 29 years, had been ill an average of 8.62 years, and had been hospitalized 6 times during the course of their illness.

Instruments

The conceptual-theoretical-empirical indicator structure for the study is presented in Table 15.1. The systems framework concepts of stress, coping, time, perception, and health were used. The middle-range theory concepts included family stressors, family coping,

TABLE 15.1 Conceptual-Theoretical-Empirical Indicator Structure for Study of Family Health in the Families of the Young Chronically Mentally Ill

Systems framework concepts	Stress	Coping	Time	Perception	Health
Theory concepts	Family stressors	Family coping	Time since diagnosis of mental illness	Family perception of client's level of health	Family health
Empirical indicators	FILE	F-COPES	Number of months from time first informed of diagnosis	PES	a. Family APGAR b. FACES III Cohesion c. FACES III Adaptability d. FES—Conflict

time since diagnosis of mental illness, family perception of the client's level of health, and family health.

Family stressors were theoretically defined as persons, objects, or events that have the potential to cause stress (King, 1981) for the family unit. The empirical indicator was the score obtained on the Family Inventory of Life Events and Changes Scale (FILE) (McCubbin, Patterson, & Wilson, 1983). The FILE functions as an index of family stress and seeks to evaluate the accumulation of normative and nonnormative family stressors.

Family coping was theoretically defined as "the constantly changing cognitive and behavioral efforts to manage specific external and internal demands that are appraised as taxing or exceeding the resources" (Lazarus & Folkman, 1984, p. 141) of the family. The operational definition of family coping was the score obtained on the Family Crisis Oriented Personal Scales (F-COPES) (McCubbin, Olson, & Larsen, 1981). The F-COPES was designed to identify problem-solving and behavioral strategies used by families in difficult situations.

The time since diagnosis of mental illness was theoretically defined as the duration of the mental illness from the time the family was first told that their member was mentally ill to the present. This term was operationally defined as the number of months from the time the family was first told of their member's mental illness to the present.

Family perception of the client's level of health was theoretically defined as the family's sense of the client's ability to function and conduct the business of living in terms of one's personal, social, and familial responsibilities. The empirical indicator for this concept was the Progress Evaluation Scale (PES) (Ihilevich, Gleser, Gritter, Kroman, & Watson, 1981). The PES was designed for an adult psychiatric population, and it focuses on the level of healthy adaptive functioning that the client is engaged in.

Family health was theoretically defined as the ability of the family unit to adjust to stressors and to function in their social roles (Frey, 1989). There were four empirical indicators for family health. The first was the Family APGAR (Smilkstein, Ashworth, & Montano, 1982), which assesses members' satisfaction with family functioning. The second empirical indicator was the FACES III Cohesion Scale (Olson, Portner, & Lavee, 1985), which was designed to measure the amount of cohesion that exists within a family unit. Cohesion was seen as essential to family functioning and thus to family health. The FACES III Adaptability Scale (Olson et al., 1985) served as the third empirical indicator. This scale was used to capture the family's ability to adjust to stressors, which is also essential to family health as defined in this study. The final empirical indicator of family health was derived from the Family Environment Scale (FES) Conflict Scale (Moos & Moos, 1981). The family's ability to manage conflict was seen as a prerequisite to being able to adjust to stressors and function in their social roles.

Procedure

The data collection procedure in this study involved several steps. First, contacts were made either by the researcher, in the case of the support groups, or by agency staff, in the case of the clinical agencies. If a family indicated an interest, the researcher followed up with a telephone call and/or letter. Families were then mailed a packet of questionnaires along with a stamped envelope for return of the materials to the researcher.

Results

The hypotheses and research questions were addressed by means of descriptive statistics, bivariate correlations, multiple correlation, and hierarchical and stepwise multiple regression. The bivariate correlations indicate that there are significant direct or indirect relationships between each of the predictor variables (family stressors, family coping, family perception of the client's level of health, and time since diagnosis) and the outcome of family health. The stepwise multiple regression equations explain between 16% and 26% of the variance in family health. Family stressors, the family coping strategy of mobilizing the family to seek out and use community resources, and the demographic variable of age of the respondent were found to be the most significant predictors of family health. Overall, the data analysis provided support for a modification of the middle-range theory of family health in the families of the young chronically mentally ill. A model of the revised middle-range theory is presented in Figure 15.2.

Discussion

The need for knowledge that is specific to the discipline of nursing has been recognized since the time of Florence Nightingale (1959). This knowledge will comprise the science of nursing and guide the practice, research, and education of the discipline. Construction of such a body of knowledge entails the delineation of metatheory, grand nursing theories, middle-range theories, and practice theories (Walker & Avant, 1988). Although the discipline has several grand theories or conceptual frameworks, there is insufficient development of middle-range theories. Several decades ago, nursing leaders, drawing from the work of Merton (1964), began calling specifically for the development of middle-range theories of nursing (Jacox, 1974). More recently, Meleis (1985) has endorsed the development of such middle-range theories as appropriate, given the fact that nursing has now identified and broadly agreed on the boundaries of nursing knowledge and nursing domain concepts.

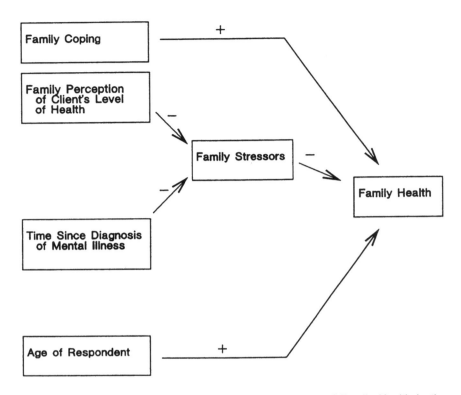

Figure 15.2. Revised Model of the Middle-Range Theory of Family Health in the Families of the Young Chronically Mentally III

Although the development of nursing theory is necessary to the establishment and expansion of the science of nursing, it is not sufficient. It is imperative that the theory be empirically tested as well (Acton, Irvin, & Hopkins, 1991; Fawcett & Downs, 1992; Silva, 1986; Silva & Sorrell, 1992). Only with such theory testing will the validity of the theory be ascertained and appropriate modifications made.

This study explored family health in the families of the young chronically mentally ill from the unique perspective of the discipline of nursing. This was accomplished by deducing a middle-range theory of family health from King's (1981) systems framework. The middle-range theory was a logical extension of, and can be traced directly back to, the work of King (1981, 1990, 1992). The resultant middle-range theory was then empirically tested. The results of the study were interpreted in light of King's framework and their implications for the proposed middle-range theory development effort.

The study results provided empirical verification, with some modifications, for the middle-range theory of family health in the families of the young chronically mentally ill. Furthermore, the research met the classic criteria set forth by Silva (1986) as necessary for adequate testing of nursing theory.

As predicted in the study hypotheses, there is a significant, positive relationship between family coping and family health. Although the total F-COPES, which was used to measure family coping, was not significantly related to family health, one of its subscales was. The F-COPES subscale of Mobilizing the Family to Acquire and Accept Help, referring to the family's ability to seek out and use community resources, was positively correlated with the outcome of family health. This relationship was consistent with King's (1981) systems framework and her application of that framework to the family (King, 1983). King (1983) asserts that when family members are unable to cope with an event or health problem, generally, they will enter the health care system and request assistance from health professionals. King (1981, 1983) spoke frequently about the role of the nurse, as a health care professional, in assisting individuals and families to cope with stressors. Given that the goal of all of nursing's endeavors, according to King (1981, 1983, 1990, 1992), is to assist individuals and families to maintain health, it appeared reasonable to assume that maximizing a family's coping skills would lead to a greater degree of health. Thus a direct relationship between family coping and family health can easily be deduced from the work of King (1981, 1983, 1990, 1992).

The specific relationship between the F-COPES Mobilize subscale and the outcome of family health can be linked to King's systems framework as well. The F-COPES Mobilize subscale assessed the ability of families to seek out and use community resources. King's (1981, 1990) definition of health includes resource use as a method to achieve and maintain health.

The significant, inverse relationship between family stressors and family health that was empirically verified indicates that as families perceived increased numbers of stressors, their level of family health was negatively affected. This finding was consistent with several of King's (1981) statements. For example, she states that "increase(s) in stress are potential predictors of subsequent illness or disease" (King, 1981, p. 98). Similarly, King (1983) suggests that "too many stressors in the family environment . . . may precipitate a crisis" (p. 182). Presumably, a crisis could lead to a lesser degree of family health at least for a period of time. Consequently, this relationship appears to be an important one for this population that can be used to guide nursing care with these families.

The significant, inverse relationship between time since diagnosis of the mental illness and family stressors can be related to King's (1981) discussion of time and stressors. She states explicitly that stress has a temporal dimension. King (1981) asserts that as a person moves from crisis to crisis there is an added dimension to stress that may increase one's stress due to past experiences or may decrease one's stress as a result of having learned to cope with past events. The inverse relationship that was empirically discovered seems to indicate that the latter scenario may be operative for the families of the young chronically mentally ill. Given this data, it appears as though family stressors may be functioning as a mediating variable between the time since diagnosis of the mental illness and the outcome of family health. Thus time since diagnosis of the mental illness has an indirect relationship to family health in the families of the young chronically mentally ill. As a result of this finding, the middle-range theory was modified from the original conceptualization.

Similarly, an indirect relationship was found between the family perception of the client's level of health and the outcome of family health. The empirical evidence suggests that family stressors function as a mediating variable between these two variables. The inverse relationship between the family perception of the client's level of health and family stressors indicates that as the client's level of health decreases, the family experiences an increased number of stressors. This relationship can be interpreted in light of King's (1981) discussion of stressors. King (1981) indicates that "people [families] respond to life events based on their unique perceptions and their interpretation of the events" (p. 98). Furthermore, she states that "a person's [family's] response to stress is influenced by . . . the meaning it has for the person [family]" (p. 98). It appears, then, that the families of the young chronically mentally ill perceive a decline in their loved one's health and functioning to be a stressful event that has negative implications for them as a family unit. The middle-range theory of family health was modified in accordance with this empirical finding as well.

It should be noted that although the empirical findings can be traced back to King's systems framework, they are also grounded in the pertinent literature pertaining to families with a mentally ill member. This provides additional validity to the middle-range theory development effort.

Summary

This study expands the science of nursing as it relates to fostering the health of the families of the young chronically mentally ill. In addition, the research adds to the theoretical base available to practitioners and suggests potential nursing interventions for these families. Further empirical testing of the middle-range theory of family health will be necessary. Such testing can assist in further explicating the complex dynamics that affect family health within this population.

References

Acton, G. J., Irvin, B. L., & Hopkins, B. A. (1991). Theory-testing research: Building the science. *Advances in Nursing Science, 14*(1), 52-61.

American Nurses Association. (1980). *ANA social policy statement.* Kansas City, MO: Author.

Chafetz, L., & Barnes, L. (1989). Issues in psychiatric caregiving. *Archives of Psychiatric Nursing, 3*(2), 61-68.

Fawcett, J. (1984). The metaparadigm of nursing: Present status and future refinements. *Image: Journal of Nursing Scholarship, 16*(3), 84-87.

Fawcett, J., & Downs, F. (1992). *The relationship of theory and research* (2nd ed.). Philadelphia: F. A. Davis.

Frey, M. A. (1989). Social support and health: A theoretical formulation derived from King's conceptual framework. *Nursing Science Quarterly*, 2(3), 138-148.

Ihilevich, D., Gleser, G. C., Gritter, G. W., Kroman, L. J., & Watson, A. S. (1981). Measuring program outcome: The Progress Evaluation Scales. *Evaluation Review*, 5(4), 451-477.

Jacox, A. (1974). Theory construction in nursing: An overview. *Nursing Research*, 23(1), 4-13.

Kane, C. (1984). The outpatient comes home: The family's response to deinstitutionalization. *Journal of Psychosocial Nursing*, 22(11), 19-25.

King, I. M. (1968). A conceptual frame of reference for nursing. *Nursing Research*, 17(1), 27-31.

King, I. M. (1971). *Toward a theory for nursing*. New York: John Wiley.

King, I. M. (1981). *A theory for nursing: Systems, concepts, process*. New York: John Wiley.

King, I. (1983). King's theory of nursing. In I. W. Clements & F. B. Roberts (Eds.), *Family health: A theoretical approach to nursing care* (pp. 177-187). New York: John Wiley.

King, I. (1990). Health as the goal for nursing. *Nursing Science Quarterly*, 3(3), 123-128.

King, I. (1992). King's theory of goal attainment. *Nursing Science Quarterly*, 5(1), 19-26.

Krauss, J. (1989). New conceptions of care, community, and chronic mental illness. *Archives of Psychiatric Nursing*, 3(5), 281-287.

Lazarus, R., & Folkman, S. (1984). *Stress, appraisal, and coping*. New York: Springer.

Lefley, H. P. (1987). Aging parents as caregivers of mentally ill adult children: An emerging social problem. *Hospital and Community Psychiatry*, 38(10), 1063-1070.

McCubbin, H. I., Olson, D. H., & Larsen, A. S. (1981). F-COPES: Family crisis oriented personal scales. In H. McCubbin & A. Thompson (Eds.), *Family assessment inventories for research and practice* (pp. 194-207). Madison: University of Wisconsin Press.

McCubbin, H. I., Patterson, J. M., & Wilson, L. (1983). FILE: Family inventory of life events and changes. In H. McCubbin & A. Thompson (Eds.), *Family assessment inventories for research and practice* (pp. 80-96). Madison: University of Wisconsin Press.

Meleis, A. (1985). *Theoretical nursing*. Philadelphia: J. B. Lippincott.

Merton, R. (1964). *Social theory and social structure* (rev. ed.). London: Free Press of Glencoe.

Moos, R. H., & Moos, B. S. (1981). *Family environment scale manual.* Palo Alto, CA: Consulting Psychologists Press.

Nightingale, F. (1959). *Notes on nursing: What it is, and what it is not.* London: Harrison & Sons.

Olson, D. H., Portner, J., & Lavee, Y. (1985). *FACES III.* St. Paul: University of Minnesota Press.

Silva, M. C. (1986). Research testing nursing theory: State of the art. *Advances in Nursing Science, 9*(1), 1-11.

Silva, M. C., & Sorrell, J. M. (1992). Testing of nursing theory: Critique and philosophical expansion. *Advances in Nursing Science, 14*(4), 12-23.

Smilkstein, G., Ashworth, C., & Montano, D. (1982). Validity and reliability of the Family APGAR as a test of family function. *Journal of Family Practice, 15*(2), 303-311.

Walker, L., & Avant, K. (1988). *Strategies for theory construction in nursing.* Norwalk, CT: Appleton & Lange.

Wilk, J. (1988). Family environments and the young chronically mentally ill. *Journal of Psychosocial Nursing, 26*(10), 15-20.

PART III

Advancing the Theory
of Goal Attainment

— 16 —

Theory of Goal Attainment

Application to Adult Orthopedic Nursing

MARTHA RAILE ALLIGOOD

$\mathbf{T}$**his chapter sets forth** King's (1981) theory of goal attainment as a structure for guiding nursing practice. King identifies the concepts of interaction, perception, communication, transaction, self, role, stress, growth and development, time, and space as those included in the theory. The chapter demonstrates the use of these concepts as a guiding focus for each phase of the nursing process. The chapter, portions of which were included in presentations at a regional conference (Smith & Alligood, 1985) and at an international conference (Alligood, 1986a, 1986b) begins with a brief presentation of King's theory of goal attainment and ideas about the nursing process that have been developed from use of the theory in practice over time.

King's Theory and the Nursing Process

Two adult clinical orthopedic cases, one acute and one chronic, will be presented using a three-dimensional view of the nursing process. The first dimension is the traditional process based on the *ANA Standards of Nursing Practice* (American Nurses Association [ANA], 1973). The second dimension uses the concepts of the theory of goal attainment (King, 1981) to focus the process. The third dimension uses King's communication process of perception, judgment, action, reaction, interaction, and transaction as a guide for the nurses' assessment of the level of communication with the client as they progress through the process. Two cases, a 17-year-old woman with multiple trauma and fractures and a 40-year-old woman with herniated nucleus pulposa, are presented using the three dimensions. Knowledge from each dimension explicates progress toward goal attainment.

The theory of goal attainment, which Imogene King derived from her conceptual framework (King, 1971, 1981), is set forth here as a structure to guide nursing practice. Whall (1989) discusses the examination of nursing conceptual models in practice and proposes that the application of nursing models in practice is an important step in their empirical examination for nursing theory development. On that basis, it could be proposed that nurses who use nursing models and theories as guides for their practice will develop a specific type of knowing about that model or theory that is impossible to achieve from contemplative exercises. Therefore, the actual application of models and theories in practice becomes particularly important for a practice discipline, such as nursing, and leads us to a new level of knowledge for theoretical development.

King (1981) has said that the focus of nursing is the care of human beings and that the goal of nursing is health. Three dynamic interacting systems—personal, interpersonal, and social—form the framework. King has specified pertinent concepts in each system and has developed her theory of goal attainment using concepts from the personal and interpersonal systems as illustrated in Table 16.1. It is important to note that with the exception of body image, the concepts of the theory of goal attainment are those of both personal and interpersonal systems. This becomes important for students of knowledge

TABLE 16.1 Concepts Included in the Model and the Theory

King's Interacting Systems	*King's Theory of Goal Attainment*
Personal system	Perception
Perception	Self
Self	Growth and development
Body image	Time
Growth and development	Space
Time	Role
Space	Interaction
Interpersonal system	Communication
Role	Transaction
Interaction	Stress
Communication	
Transaction	
Stress	
Social system	
Organization	
Power	
Authority	
Status	
Decision making	
Role	

development proposing theory testing because goal attainment might theoretically be related to either personal or interpersonal systems. King (1981) has said, "The major elements in a Theory of Goal Attainment are discovered in the interpersonal systems" (p. 142); however, the inclusion of the personal system concepts in the theory cannot be overlooked.

In this chapter, two adult clinical cases will be presented that illustrate the utility of King's theory of goal attainment in the nursing care of adult clients. The use of the theory to guide nursing practice will be made explicit in each case. King (1981) defines nursing as process of human interactions between nurse and client who communicate to set goals, explore means for achieving the goals, and then agree on the means to be used for goal attainment. Furthermore, King has said that her "theory describes the nature of nurse-client interactions that lead to achievement of goals" (p. 142). The fact that the theory specifies the outcome of nursing care or goal attainment has been identified as a strength of King's theory (Kim, 1983).

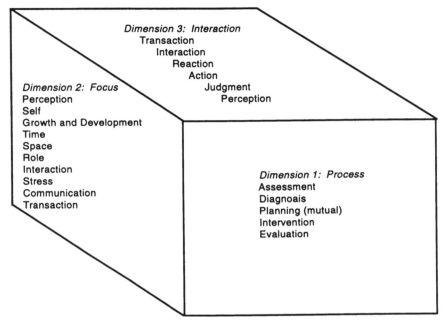

Figure 16.1.   Three-Dimensional Nursing Process Based on King

While practicing nursing with King's (1981) theory of goal attainment, three dimensions of the process have been noted. In the first
dimension, the nurse is guided by the traditional nursing process of
assessment, diagnosis, planning, treatment, and evaluation (ANA,
1973). In the second dimension, the concepts of the theory are used
as a framework (or perspective) from which to view and interact with
the client. This second dimension provides the content focus for the
process of the first dimension. King's (1981) process of human
interactions—perception, judgment, action, reaction, interaction,
and transaction (p. 145)—provides a third dimension with which one
can assess the level of communication occurring between the nurse
and the client at any point as one progresses through the nursing
process.

This three-dimensional process (Figure 16.1) was used to guide
the nursing care of an acute and a chronic orthopedic case. These
cases illustrate the utility of the three-dimensional process in guiding nursing actions toward the desired outcome of goal attainment.

Furthermore, the applications illustrate the capacity of the theory of goal attainment to structure process toward its outcome in the dynamism of the communication process and the nursing process.

Case Study 1: Lynn

The first case is a 17-year-old white Protestant female whose name is Lynn. She was an accident victim, hit by a car while riding her bicycle. She was in skeletal traction for multiple fracture of the left leg and a pelvic swing for a fractured pelvis. She also had multiple trauma with surgical repair of the vagina, rectum, and perineum. I encountered Lynn on her third hospital day. She was reportedly withdrawn, sleeping at long intervals and frequently crying. As I entered the room, the curtains were drawn and Lynn's head was turned away toward the wall. She did not look up, make eye contact, or speak to me during my first visit. This visit began the assessment phase of the first dimension; the content focus was guided by King's theory concepts for the second dimension. This theory guided content focus, clarified what was relevant and what was not (Fawcett, 1989).

Using King's concepts as the content focus for the nursing process, I began to try empathetically to understand Lynn as she might perceive her *self* in her present situation. My observation of this young woman focused on her lack of *interaction* or *communication* at this time. I noted that her *growth* and *development* status was normal for her age prior to the accident. I also learned from her chart that she was a high school senior who had already been accepted by the university of her choice for the following fall term. This information was helpful in understanding the *space* dimension. Lynn had encountered a radical assault to her space dimension in that she was riding her bicycle in her home neighborhood one day and lying in a hospital bed in traction in another city the next day. In using the third dimension, the interaction consisted of *perception, judgment,* and *action* on my part, and because there was no action (reaction) observed from Lynn, although she was conscious, I assumed perception and judgment on her part. King (1981) says that each person in the interaction makes inferences about what the other is "perceiving and thinking" because "these behaviors are not directly observable" (p. 146). It was my perception and judgment that this event had rendered her noncommunicative and, for the present time, unable to *act, react,* or *transact.* From practicing with King's (1971) framework as a guide from her earliest work, I had come to label these times, when the interaction process was seemingly halted and did not proceed, as *interaction disturbance.* My action consisted of telling her who I was and that I would be coming to see her on a regular basis for a few weeks. I also explained that I wanted us to work together and identify mutual goals for our interactions. I explained that I would be coming at the same *time* and that I wanted to talk with her when she was ready to talk with me so that we could identify mutual goals for her care. As I observed (perceived) Lynn in the context of the concepts of the theory, several questions came to mind.

The nature and extent of her injuries led me to questions regarding their impact on her normal growth and development as well as time and space in her life. For example, what impact would her hospitalization and rehabilitation have on her completion of high school and her plans for entering the university? How long would her recovery take? Also, could she anticipate normal reproductive functioning (growth and development) after the repair of her perineal and vaginal lacerations? I was told by the staff that she had not raised any of these questions so far. In fact, she had not shared her perception of what had happened, and it appeared that she (her self) was withdrawn. Her mother also voiced concern about her failure to communicate. The concepts of *stress, role,* and *time* were used to begin to understand her behavior at the present. That is, at one moment in time she had been riding her bicycle with her friends on a beautiful autumn day, and in the next moment, she was on the ground in agonizing pain. In addition to her obvious physical injuries, Lynn had a violent immediate interference in her role in life, which stressed her to the point of crisis. I concluded that the stress response to this traumatic event and the immediacy of it were overwhelming to her personal system, thus rendering her noncommunicative.

During this initial assessment, the need to support her through her experience was identified and the following nursing diagnoses were developed:

1. Impaired mobility related to fractures
2. Inability to care for self related to trauma, fractures, and stress
3. Alteration in comfort related to pain
4. Inability to interact related to stress and crisis

On the basis of my perception and judgment, and my observation of Lynn's situation, it was decided to use the nursing intervention of presence with a goal of providing support until mutual goals could be developed. Lynn remained silent through the next visit. I identified myself to her and told her how long I would stay. I told her I wanted to talk with her when she was ready and I would answer any questions she might have. Also, I told her we needed to identify mutual goals for her care and recovery.

This support, verbal and nonverbal, led through the action and reaction phases to the interaction phase of the interaction process. As Lynn began to interact, she was tearful and shared her disbelief that God could let such a thing happen to her. An additional diagnosis was identified for her care that helped target her spiritual needs and spiritual distress:

5. Spiritual distress related to, "how could God let this happen to me?"

This diagnosis was related to a short-term mutual goal to help her sort out her spiritual feelings related to the accident. Lynn was encouraged to verbalize her feelings, and she agreed to discuss her feelings with a chaplain. Later that week, her mother also asked Lynn's pastor to come for a visit. In the interaction phase, Lynn began to ask questions about the accident and asked to look at the pictures taken at the time of her accident.

Through our interaction, Lynn finally identified her goal, which was "getting ready to go home." Mutually, we agreed on that as a long-term goal. This was a turning point in Lynn's recovery. She seemed to be drawn out of her withdrawal by the nursing intervention of presence and her awareness that I was waiting for her to participate. I believe this change in Lynn's behavior occurred because I was following King's theory, which requires that mutual goals be identified before you proceed. My focus on the mutual process of goal setting seemed to engage Lynn in life again and call for her to take responsibility for her health (recovery) in concert with the nurse.

As Lynn and I began to work toward the goal of getting ready to go home, Lynn verbalized her need for information so she could better understand her condition. The following diagnosis helped identify short-term goals to facilitate the process:

6. Knowledge deficit related to extent of injuries

Lynn and I made a list of questions she wanted to ask her attending physicians. However, she still did not ask about the long-term effects of her vaginal and perineal injuries. Although I believed the topic was critical to her continued progress, I also believed we should discuss it when she was ready. I finally brought it up because she did not. Using empathy, I shared with Lynn that information about the long-term effects of her perineal injuries would be information I would want if I were in her place. Lynn immediately blurted out, "I've been wanting to talk to you about that," and began crying uncontrollably. I stayed with Lynn and, shortly, the crying ended. There was a noticeable calm and decrease in *stress*, and she verbalized feeling much better. Lynn and I put the question on the list to be discussed with the physicians.

From practicing with King, I have come to recognize these interactive breakthroughs as transactions. That is, when Lynn was able to bring what was going on in her *personal* system (intrapersonally) to the *interpersonal* system, even though it came with great difficulty, she seemed to experience reduced stress and clarity as to her role toward goal attainment. I believe the interaction process served to clarify Lynn's perception and sense of self as well as her growth and development processes in time and space. Following this breakthrough (transaction), Lynn was cheerful and seemed to have energy and enthusiasm for recovery, making plans and preparations to go home. This transaction was achieved when the short-term goal of the need to acquire knowledge was identified. Lynn was an active participant in achieving this goal through questioning the physicians and nurses who could supply the answers. Timing was critical in this process.

Shortly after Lynn began to show signs of improvement, I noticed that her mother's anxiety was increasing. I met with her mother to discuss her daughter's progress and learned that she was afraid to take Lynn home and had many questions about her care. The following diagnosis was noted for planning and intervention:

7. Ineffective family coping related to mother's anxiety

Lynn continued to make progress as she became more involved in her own care. She was placed in a body cast in preparation for discharge. A short-term goal of preparing Lynn's mother and the home for Lynn's discharge was identified mutually by the three of us. I worked very closely with Lynn's mother regarding preparation of the home for Lynn's return. Lynn's mother began to be more involved in her care, which helped reduce her anxiety and instill confidence. A hospital bed was ordered for the home, and plans were made for transfer by ambulance because Lynn was being discharged in a body cast. Arrangements were made with the local health department for nurses to visit on a regular basis. Her mother was armed with a list of phone numbers for the services she might need or persons to answer her questions. These interventions greatly reduced her anxiety by clarifying her role in her daughter's care, which also served to relieve Lynn.

On my final visit with Lynn, we both agreed that the mutual goal of getting ready to go home was attained. The following day, Lynn was discharged and accompanied by her mother in the ambulance to her home. This was possible because King's (1981) process of interaction led to transaction, facilitating goal attainment.

Case Study 2: Sarah

The second case is Sarah, a 40-year-old Jewish woman, married and mother of three, with recurring back pain. She eventually had a myelogram and spinal fusion for herniated nucleus pulposa. When I first met Sarah, she was in the hospital on bed rest and in pelvic traction for back pain. I went to answer her call light and she apologized for bothering me in that she "wasn't really sick." This interaction made me curious and led me to continue seeing Sarah. Initially, in the first dimension, I assessed her *perception* through her expressions of guilt about her inability to perform her *roles* as a mother and wife. She also was noticeably *stressed* and expressed ambivalence about the illness role related to the invisibility of the problem and a social stigma attached to "back pain" among her social circle. In regard to *time* and *space*, Sarah's stress was also related to her social schedule and the lack of time to be ill. Other second-dimension concepts besides perception, role, and stress that proved useful were *self* and *growth and development*. Sarah's discussions of her role in the family revealed a transition in the family; the children were growing up and their needs for mothering were changing.

Sarah and I moved rather quickly through *perception, judgment, action*, and *reaction* to *interaction*. She responded positively to the idea of mutual goal setting for her nursing care. I shared my observation of her reluctance to accept the illness role and she agreed for us to work on that area. The following nursing diagnoses were identified from the assessment and mutually agreed on with Sarah:

1. Alteration in health maintenance related to her inability to accept the illness and the illness role
2. Alteration in comfort related to back pain
3. Disturbance in self-concept related to family transition
4. Disturbance in role relationships related to role deprivation and social isolation
5. Ineffective coping related to stress intolerance

After meeting with Sarah a few times, I sensed my own frustration at her inability to believe there really was a problem with her back. So I made arrangements for a viewing box and her films to be brought to her room. When Sarah saw the herniated nucleus pulposa on the film, she began to cry. When her crying ended, her stress was noticeably decreased and she said she felt better. She began to be able to accept the illness role, relinquish her mother and wife responsibilities for a time, and admit she needed help through this experience. As in the previous case presentation, crying accompanied a breakthrough that not only reduced stress but also clarified the role that Sarah should take in her own progress toward health. Interacting about that realization was a *transaction* for Sarah, and she expressed relief in accepting the illness role and said she was now ready to have her surgery.

Sarah went home for 2 weeks of bed rest and then returned to the hospital for surgery. The surgery and postoperative period were not remarkable. Sarah did well and was discharged home. I made a home visit and found Sarah stressed once again. We explored what was happening to cause her feelings. Through the interaction she identified being in her home "space" and unable to fulfill her roles as a problem, but there also seemed to be something else bothering her. In listening to Sarah's recount of the events leading up to and following her surgery, the idea of loss came to me and I shared my idea with her. When I mentioned loss, it was as though the flood gates were opened and Sarah began to cry and sob, telling me that she felt foolish about her small loss, but she had lost a part of her body and it was gone forever. The expression of these feelings of loss, through interaction, led Sarah to observable stress reduction and transaction, once again, in that it moved her quickly through recovery. From that point on, she reorganized her life and adjusted to the changes in her wife/mother/society roles with a perception of self appropriate for the current time. I returned to terminate our relationship, at which time I removed Sarah's stitches, and we enjoyed a delightful lunch together.

Research Implications

Each of the cases presented illustrates the value of the perspective afforded by King's (1981) theory of goal attainment. Whereas the physical condition of the client was an essential element in each case, use of the theory of goal attainment and the three-dimensional process led to interaction through which the broader meaning of the illness experience for each client was revealed. In this broader holistic context, the transactions occurred, when the clients seemingly experienced a breakthrough, which then led to the desired nursing outcome or goal attainment.

These cases highlight the need for clinical research to develop a better understanding of the phenomena of transaction. In each case, and twice in the second one, the progress toward goal attainment seems blocked or hindered by the client's inability to identify or verbalize that which seems to be imperative to her progress. With identity and verbalization, something dramatic occurs that needs to be studied. I have understood these breakthroughs as transactions because they seem to be associated with rapid movement toward goal achievement once they have occurred. Possible research questions might include the following:

1. What is the nature of the reluctance or inability of clients to identify or verbalize their goals?
2. What is the relationship between expression of emotion (crying) and the timing of clients' ability to identify or verbalize their problem or goal? In other words, does emotional expression precede, accompany, or follow the breakthrough?
3. How do clients describe the experience of these breakthroughs (transactions) that lead to goal attainment?
4. Is the progress toward goal attainment impeded intrapersonally or interpersonally? In other words, is the interaction disturbance a function of the intrapersonal client system, the interpersonal (nurse-client) relationship, or both?
5. What is the relationship between interaction disturbance and breakthroughs that lead to transaction and goal attainment?

Summary

In this chapter I have presented King's (1981) theory of goal attainment, which she derived from her interacting systems framework. King's perspective amplifies the nurse-client interaction as was presented in a three-dimensional nursing process format. First, the traditional nursing process dimension; second, the concepts, content, and focus dimension of the theory of goal attainment; and third, the human interaction dimension for evaluation of the communication process.

The three-dimensional nursing process format presented in this chapter extends King's ideas of the interface of these processes (King,

1990) and addresses the criticism of limited clinical utility of her theory in practice to guide the process or specify interventions (Meleis, 1991). The two cases presented illustrate utility of the theory of goal attainment as a guide in nursing practice for assessment, diagnosis, and intervention. Furthermore, the use of the actual concepts of the theory as the content focus of assessment, the second dimension of the process presented in this chapter, demonstrates how the theory does offer guidelines for interventions and how the interventions emerge from the nursing diagnoses. This strength of King's (1981) interacting systems framework and theory of goal attainment as a framework for nursing process has also been noted by Evans (1991), who has proposed an assessment format that includes five concepts of King's (1981) theory. Both Evans's format and the one presented in this chapter recognize the importance of allowing the very concepts of the theory to provide the content focus of the mutual process with the client.

Two cases, Lynn (a patient with acute multiple trauma) and Sarah (a patient with chronic back pain), were presented. These cases illustrate the utility of King's (1981) interacting systems framework and the theory of goal attainment as a guide for nursing practice. A particular benefit of King's (1981) perspective is its alignment with the traditional nursing process, which can facilitate understanding of the framework and theory among practicing nurses. Furthermore, the use of the traditional nursing process leads to correlation with the *Standards of Nursing Practice* (ANA, 1973), and this relationship facilitates quality assurance efforts based on nursing standards. It is interesting to note that in the new *ANA Standards of Clinical Nursing Practice* (ANA, 1991), an additional step, "outcome identification," has been added after nursing diagnosis and before planning. Although this addition may prove useful with other models, King's emphasis on mutual goal setting incorporated outcome identification from the beginning (King, 1971, 1981).

Finally, the value of King's (1981) framework of interacting systems and the theory of goal attainment as guides for nursing research has been identified. Practicing with King's theory, as illustrated by the cases presented here, highlights the need to study and better understand the impact of King's human interactions process on client outcomes.

References

Alligood, M. (1986a). The goal of transaction: Application of King's theory as a guide for nursing practice with adults [abstract]. In *Proceedings of the Nursing Theory Congress, Theoretical pluralism: Direction for a practice discipline* (pp. 93-94). Toronto, Ontario: Ryerson School of Nursing.

Alligood, M. (Speaker). (1986b). The goal of transaction: Application of King's theory as a guide for nursing practice with adults. On *Papers— Imogene King's framework* (cassette recording No. 860819-121). Markham, Ontario: Audio Archives of Canada.

American Nurses Association. (1973). *ANA standards of nursing practice.* (1973). Kansas City, MO: Author.

American Nurses Association. (1991). *ANA standards of clinical nursing practice.* Kansas City, MO: Author.

Evans, C. (1991). *Imogene King: A conceptual framework for nursing.* Newbury Park, CA: Sage.

Fawcett, J. (1989). *Conceptual models of nursing* (2nd ed.). Philadelphia: F. A. Davis.

Kim, H. S. (1983). *The nature of theoretical thinking in nursing.* Norwalk, CT: Appleton-Century-Crofts.

King, I. (1971). *Toward a theory for nursing.* New York: John Wiley.

King, I. (1981). *A theory for nursing: Systems, concepts, process.* New York: John Wiley.

King, I. (1990). King's conceptual framework and theory of goal attainment. In M. Parker (Ed.), *Nursing theories in practice* (pp. 73-84). New York: National League for Nursing.

Meleis, A. (1991). *Theoretical nursing* (2nd ed.). New York: J. B. Lippincott.

Smith, D., & Alligood, M. (1985, October). *Matching nursing models to clinical practice.* Paper presented at the King session conducted at the Region 7 Meeting of Sigma Theta Tau International, Atlanta, GA.

Whall, A. (1989). Nursing science: The process and the products. In J. Fitzpatrick & A. Whall (Eds.), *Conceptual models of nursing* (pp. 1-14). Norwalk, CT: Appleton & Lange.

17

Perceptual Congruency
Between Clients and Nurses

Testing King's Theory of Goal Attainment

DOROTHY FROMAN

The nature of nursing requires frequent interactions between clients and nurses. The nurse, as the helping person, must understand clients from their own frame of reference. A factor hypothesized by King (1981) as influential in nurse-client interactions was perception. This chapter presents a study that examined perceptual congruency between clients and nurses regarding the illness situation, nursing care, and client satisfaction with care.

Statement of the Problem

The literature that addresses nurse-client perceptual congruency is limited. A study by Davies and Peters (1983) examined nurse-client perceptions of client stress related to hospitalization. The study results indicated a difference between the ratings of the nurse-client pairs. A study by Freeman and Hefferin (1984) showed incongruency between nurse-client perceptions of client reactions to hospitalization. Jennings and Muhlenkamp (1981) reported a statistically significant discrepancy in perception of client affective states by nurse-client pairs.

Theoretical Framework

A clear conceptualization of the nature of nurse-client interactions was seen as an important component in the development of nursing knowledge. King (1981) conceptualized nursing as operating within three interacting systems—the personal, interpersonal, and social. King (1981) derived a theory of goal attainment from the interpersonal component of her framework. The theory proposes that during nurse-client interactions, information is shared and transactions occur in which the values, needs, and wants of each person are shared and the perceptions of the nurse, client, and the situation influence the interaction. The theory of goal attainment describes the nature of the nurse-client encounter and provides a theoretical base for the nursing process.

Purpose

The study was designed as exploratory, correlational research at the factor-relating level of theory development. The specific concepts of perception and transaction from King's (1981) theory of goal attainment were examined. The purpose of the study was to explore the degree of perceptual congruency between clients and nurses related to the illness situation and the nursing care required. The study was linked to the developing knowledge base of nursing through the exploration of a proposition modified from the theory of goal attainment—namely, that perceptual congruency between nurse and client facilitates transactions leading to goal attainment and effective nursing care.

Research Questions

1. Is there a difference between clients' and nurses' perceptions of the clients' illness situation and nursing care required?
2. Is there a relationship between client and nurse perceptual congruency and client satisfaction with nursing care?

The study hypothesis was, *The greater the degree of perceptual congruency between nurse and client related to the illness situation and nursing care required, the greater the degree of goal attainment or satisfaction with nursing care.*

The study proposition was, *The presence of perceptual congruency between nurse and client influences the occurrence of transaction leading to goal attainment or effective nursing care.*

Definitions

1. Illness situation: An imbalance in the person's biological, psychological, or social system as perceived and experienced by the person (King, 1981, p. 5).
2. Transaction: The process whereby the nurse and client share their frame of reference about the illness situation in order to work toward goal attainment of effective nursing care and satisfactory client outcome (King, 1981, p. 147).
3. Perceptual congruency: The degree of similarity between nurse and client perception of the understanding of the illness situation and nursing care required as measured by a research-designed questionnaire.
4. Client satisfaction: The degree of satisfaction with nursing care as perceived by the client and measured operationally by the Patient Satisfaction With Care Scale (Hefferin, 1979).

Method

The study was conducted on the medical and surgical units of three urban community-based hospitals. A nonprobability convenience sample of 40 matched nurse-client pairs was used for the study. The criteria for selection into the study sample for the client group were as follows: (a) must be aged 18 years and older; (b) must have a medical or surgical diagnosis; (c) must be able to read, write, and speak English; (d) must be on a medical or surgical unit for a minimum of 3 days; and (e) must be willing to participate in the study. The criteria for inclusion in the nurse group were as follows: (a) must be a registered nurse, (b) must have interacted with the client for a minimum of three shifts either cumulative or consecutive, and (c) must be willing to participate in the study. The client sample consisted of 26 (65%) females and 14 (35%) males, with 50% (20) being 51 years of age and over. Grade school was the highest education level attained by 55% (22) of the sample. Medical treatment was the reason for hospitalization for 60% (24) of the sample, with 70% (28) of the clients staying in the hospital for 11 days and over. The registered nurse sample was 97.5% (39) female and 2.5% (1) male, with 47.5% (19) of the sample being 20 to 29 years of age and 97.5% (39) diploma-nursing prepared.

Measurement Instruments

The Patient Satisfaction With Care Scale (Hefferin, 1979) was used to examine client satisfaction with nursing care. This questionnaire was designed to examine the effect of mutual goal setting on client health outcome and satisfaction with nursing care. Cronbach's alpha was used to estimate the reliability of the questionnaire for the study. Results of 0.8779 indicated that the instrument was reliable in this study.

The Perceptual Congruency Questionnaire, the researcher-designed instrument, was used to measure nurse-client perceptual congruency of the illness situation and nursing care required. The questions were grounded in the steps of the nursing process. Involvement of the client and validation of perceptions was seen as an integral part of the nursing process (Daubenmire & King, 1973; Griffith & Christensen, 1982; LaMonica, 1985; Neuman, 1982; Orque, Bloch, & Monrroy, 1983; Pasquali, Arnold, & DeBasio, Alesi, 1985; Yura & Walsh, 1983). The questionnaire is available from the author.

The questions were separated into three categories: perception of the illness, perception of mutual goal setting, and perception of information communicated to reflect the proposition examined in the study and King's (1981) theory of goal attainment.

Cronbach's alpha indicated that the questionnaire items were reliable in this study (0.9130: clients; 0.8456: nurses).

Procedure

The nurse-client pairs were chosen in consultation with the head nurse or designate. The consent form ensured that subjects' rights were protected. Data were collected on day and evening shifts, 7 days of the week. Questionnaires were administered in a private area, collected immediately on completion, and coded numerically to ensure anonymity.

Data Analysis

Descriptive statistics, frequencies, and measures of central tendency were generated on the study variables. The Kolmogrov-Smirnov goodness-of-fit test was used to determine a normal test distribution. The Sign test; the Wilcoxon matched-pairs, signed-ranks test; and paired t test were used to examine differences in responses. The Pearson correlation coefficient, Kendall coefficient of concordance, Spearman correlation coefficient tests, and scattergrams were used to examine relationships. Multiple analysis of variance (MANOVA) was used to determine the influence of selected demographic variables on the study variables. The reliability of the study instruments was determined by the Cronbach's alpha.

Study Results

The descriptive statistics generated on the perceptual congruency questionnaire indicated that a small majority ($n = 23$, 57.5%) of the nurse-client pairs were congruent in their responses. The first category of the questionnaire, Perception of the Illness Situation, asked questions that would be included in a basic nursing history assessment. Although congruency was shown on the majority of the items, some interesting data were elicited. Table 17.1 depicts the nurses' responses to the questions.

The majority of the nurses (n = 22, 52.5%) were either uncertain or did not understand what clients believed caused their illness to occur. Twelve (30%) were uncertain or did not understand how the client's family had reacted to the illness. Twenty (50%) were uncertain or did not understand how the client had coped with previous illness experience. Fifteen (37.5%) were unsure how the illness had affected the client's working life. Nine (22%) were uncertain about or did not understand what was the client's major concern.

The second category, Perception of Mutual Goal Setting, focused on the planning and implementation of nursing care. The results (shown in Table 17.2) of the nurse-client responses showed a difference between the pairs. Ten (25%) of the nurses did not understand or were uncertain of the client's personal preferences about nursing care or the client's need to make decisions about care. Eight (20%) of the nurses were uncertain or did not understand what kind of nursing care the client felt would be most helpful or what was expected of the nurses. Fourteen (34.5%) nurses were uncertain or did not understand how the clients felt about the nursing actions developed for the client.

Category 3, Perception of Information Communicated, focused on basic health teaching to clients. The differences between the nurse-client pairs were less obvious in this set of questions; however, the responses indicated some incongruencies (see Table 17.3).

Of the nurses, 20% (8) were uncertain or did not understand what the client needed to know about the medications he or she was taking; 45% (8) were unsure of the client's need for knowledge about activities at home. Nine (25%) were uncertain or did not understand what the clients needed to know about tests and procedures, and 14 (35%) of the nurses were uncertain or did not understand the client's need for knowledge about caring for self at home.

TABLE 17.1 Frequency Distribution (in percentages, means, and standard deviations) of Nurse Responses[a] to the Perceptual Congruency Questionnaire—Category 1: Perception of the Illness Situation ($n = 40$)

Item	Percentages			Mean	Standard Deviation
	Well Understood, Understood	Uncertain	Somewhat Understood, Not at All Understood		
What your patient believes caused the illness to occur	47.5	22.5	30.0	3.275	1.154
What your patient is most concerned about	77.5	17.5	5.0	4.000	0.816
How your patient's family has reacted to the illness	47.5	2.5	27.5	3.250	1.214
How your patient's illness has affected everyday activities	85.0	5.0	10.0	4.050	0.959
How your patient has managed previous experience with illness	50.0	32.5	17.5	3.400	1.033
How your patient feels about being in hospital at this time	95.0	0	5.0	4.200	0.687
How this illness has affected your patient's working life	57.5	30.0	7.5	3.632	0.883
The most important result your patient hopes to achieve from treatment	77.5	12.5	10.0	3.900	0.955

a. How well were you able to understand your patient's view of these items?

229

TABLE 17.2 Frequency Distribution (in percentages, means, and standard deviations) of Nurse Responses[a] to the Perceptual Congruency Questionnaire—Category 2: Perception of Mutual Goal Setting (n = 40)

Item	Percentages			Mean	Standard Deviation
	Well Understood, Understood	Uncertain	Somewhat Understood, Not at All Understood		
What kind of nursing care your patient feels will be most helpful	80.0	12.5	7.5	4.000	0.847
How your patient feels about the nursing actions developed for his or her care	65.0	32.0	3.0	3.875	0.822
What your patient feels he or she should do to help himself or herself get better	72.5	7.5	20.0	3.700	1.067
What your patient expects you to do for him or her while in the hospital	80.0	7.5	12.5	4.000	0.961
Your patient's need to make decisions about his or her own care	72.5	17.5	7.5	3.949	0.887
What your patient's personal preferences about his or her nursing care are	75.0	12.5	12.5	3.900	0.955

a. How well were you able to understand your patient's view of these items?

TABLE 17.3 Frequency Distribution (in percentages, means, and standard deviations) of Nurse Responses[a] to the Perceptual Congruency Questionnaire—Category 3: Perception of Information Communicated ($n = 40$)

Item	Percentages			Mean	Standard Deviation
	Well Understood, Understood	Uncertain	Somewhat Understood, Not at All Understood		
Your patient's need for a comfortable environment	92.5	2.5	2.5	4.359	0.668
What your patient needs to know about his or her illness	77.5	10.0	12.5	3.825	0.874
What your patient needs to know about the medications he or she is taking	80.0	15.0	5.0	4.015	0.800
What your patient needs to know about tests and procedures	77.5	7.5	15.0	3.925	1.071
What your patient needs to know about caring for himself or herself at home	62.5	30.0	5.0	3.846	0.875
What your patient needs to know about the type and amount of activity he or she should have at home	55.0	30.0	15.0	3.575	0.958
What your patient needs to know about the type of diet he or she should be following at home	65.0	22.5	10.0	3.872	0.978

a. How well were you able to understand your patient's view of these items?

The responses to the patient satisfaction with care questionnaire were generally positive (see Table 17.4). The variation in responses indicated that clients were able to express some dissatisfaction.

Fourteen clients (35%) were not satisfied with the encouragement they had received to have a say or voice in the health care services provided. Nineteen (47.5%) of the clients were not satisfied with the quality of health care teaching received from their nurse. Eleven (27.5%) were not satisfied with the encouragement they had received from their nurse to identify their own health goals or evaluate their own health progress.

The first research question asked if there was a difference between clients' and nurses' perceptions of the client's illness situation and nursing care required. The results of the nonparametric Sign test ($r = 2.433$, $p = .01$) and the Wilcoxon matched-pairs, signed-rank test ($r = 2.26$, $p = .02$) indicated a difference in the responses of the clients and nurses. The results of the parametric paired t test indicated that there was a difference between the mean responses of the clients and nurses ($t = 1.79$, $p = .04$). Pearson correlation coefficient results ($r = .0719$, $p = .330$) indicated a lack of relationship between nurses' and clients' perceptual congruencies. A scattergram was generated to further check the results. No significant relationship was shown.

The second research question asked if there was a relationship between client perceptual congruency and client satisfaction with care. The two questionnaires, perceptual congruency and patient satisfaction with care, provided the data to examine the concepts from the theory of goal attainment pertinent to the study. Pearson correlation coefficient results showed a moderately strong relationship ($r = .4334$, $p = .003$). The results were supported by the scattergram results and the Spearman rank correlation results of $r = .4890$. Thus a significant relationship was shown.

The study hypothesis—that the greater the degree of perceptual congruency between nurse and client related to the illness situation and nursing care required, the greater the degree of goal attainment or satisfaction with nursing care—was statistically supported. A significant relationship was indicated by both the Pearson correlation coefficient results ($r = .4344$, $p = .003$) and the Spearman correlation

TABLE 17.4 Frequency Distribution (in percentages, means, and standard deviations) of Client Responses[a] on Patient Satisfaction With Care Questionnaire ($n = 40$)

Item	Percentages		Mean	Standard Deviation
	Always/ Mostly Satisfied	Occasionally/ Not at All Satisfied		
The general information you have been given by your nurse about your overall health condition	85.0	15.0	4.175	1.259
The ways you have been shown by your nurse for assessing your own current health problems and needs	80.0	20.0	4.075	1.309
Your being encouraged by your nurse to identify your own health care goals	72.5	27.5	3.875	1.399
The information you have been given by your nurse about the purpose of nursing care activities	75.0	25.0	3.950	1.484
The ways you have been shown to evaluate the degree of your own health care progress	72.5	27.5	3.800	1.522
The quality of health care teaching you have received from your nurse	52.5	47.5	3.150	1.733
The encouragement you have received to have a say or voice in the health care services provided	65.0	35.0	3.525	1.679
The explanations you have been given about the responsibilities you have in your own health care	72.5	27.5	3.725	1.519
The ways in which your nurse treated you as an individual person with special health problems and needs	95.0	5.0	4.675	0.764
The ways you have been shown to identify and to plan for coping with your own health problems and needs in the future	60.0	40.0	3.375	1.779

a. How satisfied are you with these items.

233

results $(r = .4980, p = .001)$. The results provided support for the study proposition as well.

Discussion

This study was designed to explore the concepts of perception and transaction as described in King's (1981) theory of goal attainment. There were no studies in the literature that examined perceptual congruency between nurse-client dyads regarding the illness situation and nursing care required.

The framework for the study was the theory of goal attainment as proposed by King (1981). Perception is defined within King's framework as "each human being's representation of reality . . . a process of organizing, interpreting and transforming information from sensory data and memory" (King, 1981, p. 24).

Transactions are defined as "a process of interaction in which human beings communicate with the environment to achieve goals that are valued. Transactions are goal-directed human behaviors" (King, 1981, p. 82).

The study results indicated that the perceptions of the nurse-client pairs regarding the illness situation and nursing care required were dissimilar. The paired t test showed a difference between the mean responses of the clients and nurses $(t = 1.79, p = .04)$. The correlation tests did not show evidence of a relationship between the nurse-client scores $(r = .472, p = .386)$.

The results could have been influenced by a number of factors. One of these factors may have been the design of the questionnaire. The items on the perceptual congruency questionnaire were designed within the context of the theory of goal attainment. This theory proposes that during nurse-client interactions "information is shared, mutual goals are set, and clients are asked to participate in decisions about the means to achieve the goals" (King, 1981, p. 176).

The items on the perceptual congruency questionnaire may have sought information not readily available if nurses have not obtained assessment data, involved clients in decision making, and provided basic health teaching. The results suggested that validation by nurses with their clients about the means to achieve client goals may occur minimally in actual practice. The nursing process had been endorsed by the nursing profession and has been the basis of nursing education programs and nursing practice since the mid-1970s (Manitoba Association of Registered Nurses, 1981). However, as Farrell and Tamblyn (1986) have pointed out, there is evidence of dissonance between the acceptance and application of the nursing process by practicing nurses. The difference in nurse-client perceptual congruency may have been related to the implementation of the nursing process in actual practice.

The results of the correlation tests showed a moderately strong relationship between high nurse-client perceptual congruency scores and satisfaction with care ($r = .4334, p = .003$). It would appear that the clients who believed that their nurse understood them were more satisfied with their care than were the clients who felt that their nurse did not understand them as well. This result underlines the importance of promoting understanding between clients and their nurses in order to reach positive health outcomes.

The frequency distribution indicated that the general trend of the scores on the satisfaction with care questionnaire was positive. This result was not unexpected. The literature has shown that the results on the satisfaction with care questionnaire tend to be high scores (French, 1981; LaMonica, Oberst, Madea, & Wolfe, 1986; Oberst, 1984; Ventura, Fox, Corley, & Mercurio, 1982). The need to give socially acceptable answers may have contributed to the generally high scores.

It should also be noted that the client sample was composed mainly of middle-aged and older females. The literature has shown that older clients are consistently more satisfied with their hospital care (Abdellah & Levine, 1957; Locker & Dunt, 1978; Nelson-Wernick, Currey, & Paylor, 1981; Ware, Davies-Avery, & Stewart, 1978; Watterson, 1971). The adoption of the passive role by the clients may have contributed to the generally positive scores. Tagliacozzo and Mauksch (1972) proposed that clients often feel "helpless" in evaluating the knowledge, skills, and competence of caregivers and are thus reluctant to express their opinions even when they are certain of their judgment ability.

The study results provided support that validation with and involvement of the client are important components of effective nursing practice and client satisfaction with care. Incorporation of the findings in nursing practice might lead to increased satisfaction for both clients and nurses.

The study hypothesis—that the greater the degree of perceived perceptual congruency between nurse and client related to the illness situation and nursing care required, the greater the degree of goal attainment or satisfaction with care—was statistically supported. This finding provides support for King's (1981) theory of goal attainment. It appears that perception by clients that nurses understand them can influence the clients' satisfaction with care. The statistical results also provided support for the study proposition that the presence of perceptual congruency between nurse and client influences the occurrence of transaction leading to goal attainment or effective nursing care. It appears that if information is shared and validated with clients and clients are allowed to participate in decision making related to their care, their satisfaction with care is increased. This finding pointed out the importance for the nurse to understand the client's perception of the illness situation, along with the importance of understanding the client's perceptions regarding health teaching, and reinforced the importance of involvement of clients in all phases of the nursing process.

Because the study results raised a considerable number of questions about the use of the nursing process by nurses, an important finding of the study was the need for empirical validation of the nursing process.

There were also implications in the study for nurse administrators. Do current staffing levels and staffing practices allow for meaningful interactions between clients and nurses?

The results of the study provide an impetus for further research into the methods of delivering nursing services. A qualitative study to explore whether there are barriers in the health care system in the provision of effective nursing care needs to be initiated. Investigation of mutual goal setting in a variety of clinical settings may provide a more effective method of nursing care delivery.

Conclusion

This investigation provided evidence to support perceptual congruency between clients and nurses as an important component of nursing interactions. In addition, nurse-client perceptual congruency appeared to be an indicator of client satisfaction with care. The results provided support for the concepts of perception and transaction in the nurse-client encounter as outlined in King's theory of goal attainment. Through research, nursing can continue to strive for improvement in nursing practice.

References

Abdellah, F., & Levine, E. (1957). Developing a measure of patient and personal satisfaction with nursing care. *Nursing Research, 5*(3), 100-108.

Daubenmire, M. J., & King, I. (1973). Nursing process models: A systems approach. *Nursing Outlook, 21,* 512-517.

Davies, A., & Peters, M. (1983). Stresses of hospitalization in the elderly: Nurses' and patients' perceptions. *Journal of Advanced Nursing, 8,* 99-105.

Farrell, P., & Tamblyn, R. (1986). *The cognitive process of the practicing nurse.* Unpublished manuscript, Winnipeg, Manitoba.

Freeman, C., & Hefferin, E. (1984, April). Are you out of touch with your patients? *RN,* pp. 51-53.

French, K. (1981). Methodological considerations in hospital patient opinion surveys. *International Journal of Nursing Studies, 18*(1), 7-32.

Griffith, J., & Christensen, P. (1982). *Nursing process application of theories, frameworks, and models.* Toronto, Ontario: C. V. Mosby.

Hefferin, E. (1979). Health goal setting: Patient nurse collaboration at VA facilities. *Military Medicine, 144,* 814-822.

Jennings, B., & Muhlenkamp, P. (1981). Systematic misperception: Oncology patients' self-reported affective states and their care-givers' perceptions. *Cancer Nursing, 4*(6),485-489.

King, I. M. (1981). *A theory for nursing: Systems, concepts, process.* New York: John Wiley.

LaMonica, E. (1985). *The humanistic nursing process.* Monterey, CA: Wadsworth.

LaMonica, E., Oberst, M., Madea, A., & Wolfe, M. (1986). Development of a patient satisfaction scale. *Research in Nursing and Health, 9,* 43-50.

Locker, D., & Dunt, D. (1978). Theoretical and methodological issues in sociological studies of consumer satisfaction with medical care. *Social Science and Medicine, 12,* 283-292.

Manitoba Association of Registered Nurses. (1981). *Standards of nursing care.* Winnipeg, Manitoba: Author.

Nelson-Wernick, E., Currey, H., & Paylor, P. (1981, Winter). Patient perception of medical care. *Health Care Management Review,* pp. 65-72.

Neuman, B. (1982). *The Neuman systems model.* Norwalk, CT: Appleton-Century-Crofts.

Oberst, M. (1984). Patient's perception of care measurement of quality and satisfaction. *Cancer, 53*(10), 2366-2373.

Orque, M., Bloch, B., & Monrroy, L. (1983). *Ethnic nursing care: A multicultural approach.* Toronto, Ontario: C. V. Mosby.

Pasquali, E., Arnold, H., DeBasio, N., & Alelsi, E. (1985). *Mental health nursing: A holistic approach* (2nd ed.). Toronto, Ontario: C. V. Mosby.

Tagliacozzo, D., & Mauksch, H. (1972). The patient's view of the patient's role. In E. Jaco (Ed.), *Patients, physicians and illness* (2nd ed., pp. 172-185). New York: Free Press.

Ventura, M., Fox, R., Corley, M., & Mercurio, S. (1982). A patient satisfaction measure as a criterion to evaluate primary nursing. *Nursing Research, 31*(4), 226-230.

Ware, J., Davies-Avery, A., & Stewart, A. (1978, February). The measurement and meaning of patient satisfaction. *Health and Medical Care Services Review,* pp. 1-16.

Watterson, R. (1971, February). Determining public attitudes. *Hospitals,* pp. 57-59.

Yura, H., & Walsh, M. (1983). *The nursing process* (4th ed.). New York: Appleton-Century-Crofts.

18

Use of King's Theory of
Goal Attainment to Promote
Adolescents' Health Behavior

KATHLEEN M. HANNA

Promoting healthy behavior is important during the developmental period of adolescence, a time known for risk-taking behaviors that have the potential to jeopardize adolescents' health (Baumrind, 1987). Reduction of adolescents' risk-taking behaviors could prevent many of their health problems (Millstein, 1989).

Theoretically based interventions are needed to influence adolescents' health behavior. King's (1981) theory of goal attainment provides a means for nursing prescriptions to change adolescents' health behavior.

The purpose of this chapter is to describe the use of King's (1981) theory of goal attainment to promote healthy behavior among adolescents. First, the theory of goal attainment as a means for changing behavior will be discussed. King's (1981) theory will be augmented in the area of perceptions by the Health Belief Model (Rosenstock,

LEVEL OF THEORY   CONCEPTS

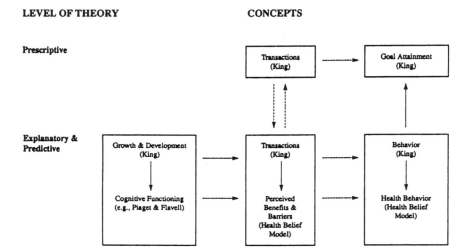

Figure 18.1. Level of Theories and Relationships Between Concepts of King's Theory, the Health Belief Model, and Cognitive Developmental Theory
NOTE: Arrows with solid lines denote deduction from abstract to more specific concepts. Arrows with broken lines denote the influence of concepts on other concepts.

1966). The area of nurse-client transactions by King (1981) will be supported by influential communications as delineated by Kasch (1986), Kasch and Knutson (1985), and Kasch and Lisnek (1984). The influence of growth and development, specifically cognitive development, on perceptions will support the need for nurse-client transactions. Finally, testing the theory of goal attainment with a population of female adolescents will be discussed. The discussion will emphasize the proposition and hypothesis that were tested. The nurse-client transaction involved oral contraceptive perceptions. The goal to be attained was oral contraceptive adherence.

Figure 18.1 delineates the relationships between the theories and concepts that will be discussed. King's (1981) theory of goal attainment provides the more abstract concepts of transactions and goal attainment. At the prescriptive theory level, the influential relationship between the concepts is this: Transactions lead to goal attainment (King, 1981). At the explanatory and predictive theory level are the concepts of growth and development, perceptions, and behavior as delineated in King's (1981) systems framework. The influential relationships between these concepts are these: Growth and development influence perceptions and perceptions influence behavior (King, 1981). From King's (1981) abstract concepts of growth and development, perceptions, and behavior, the less abstract concepts of cognitive functioning, perceived benefits and barriers, and health behavior are deduced. The influential relationships between these concepts are these: Cognitive functioning influences perceived benefits and barriers, and perceived benefits and barriers influence health behavior.

Theory of Goal Attainment

King's (1981) theory of goal attainment focuses on the interpersonal system of the nurse and client. The interpersonal system is characterized by interactions between the personal systems of the nurse and client. Transaction is the type of nurse-client interaction that influences behavior. Transaction is the process of exchanging and negotiating between nurse and client and involves perceptions of the nurse and client in the interaction. When the nurse and client have a transaction, goal attainment or a mutually desired behavioral outcome is achieved.

King's (1981) concept of transaction is supported by the concept of influential communication, as delineated by Kasch (1986), Kasch and Knutson (1985), and Kasch and Lisnek (1984). Influential communication is based on the client's subjective perspective and involves modification of perceptions. The uniqueness and individuality of the client is emphasized in influential communications between the nurse and client. Behavioral change occurs through influential communication.

Congruency exists between influential communication (Kasch, 1986; Kasch & Knutson, 1985; Kasch & Lisnek, 1984) and transactions (King, 1981). Both influential communication and transactions focus on the individual's subjective perspective or perceptions. Furthermore, for both influential communication and transactions, the individual's perceptions are the center of a dynamic process that influences behavior or goal attainment (a mutually desired behavior).

The proposition that behavioral change occurs through influential communication supports King's (1981) proposition that transactions lead to goal attainment.

Perceptions

Perceptions are an integral aspect of transactions. King (1981) defines perception as "each person's subjective world of experience" (p. 146) and as "a process of organizing, interpreting, and transforming information from sense data and memory" (p. 24).

Perceptions as described in King's (1981) theory can be augmented by perceptions delineated in the Health Belief Model (Rosenstock, 1966). The Health Belief Model (Rosenstock, 1966) proposes that perceptions influence behavior and that one's environment influences these perceptions. Perceptions of susceptibility, seriousness, benefits, and barriers constitute the cluster of beliefs involved in influencing health behavior. These perceptions have been defined as (a) perceived susceptibility as the subjective risk of contracting the condition, (b) perceived seriousness as the belief about the seriousness of the condition, (c) perceived benefits as the belief about the availability as well as the effectiveness of the health behavior, and (d) perceived barriers as the belief about the negative aspects of the health behavior (Rosenstock, 1966, pp. 99-100).

These perceptions serve as variables within a decision-making process. Perceived susceptibility and seriousness together are a health threat that provides the individual with the energy or readiness for action. Perceived benefits to the health behavior are weighed against perceived barriers and a decision is made about the health behavior.

Empirical support for the Health Belief Model (Rosenstock, 1966) is suggested from findings of numerous studies. A positive relationship between health behavior and perceived susceptibility, seriousness, and benefits has been reported, whereas a negative relationship has been reported between perceived barriers and health behavior (Becker, 1976; Haynes, 1976; Janz & Becker, 1984; Mikhail, 1981; Redeker, 1988). Of these relationships between health perceptions and behavior, the most empirical support was for perceived barriers inhibiting health behavior (Janz & Becker, 1984).

The majority of studies suggesting a relationship between perceptions and behavior have been retrospective. With retrospective data, findings need to be interpreted with caution because these perceptions may not precede the behavior and the behavior may precede the perceptions. A limited number of studies have been prospective, and even fewer studies have been experimental. However, the findings of these limited studies support that perceptions do influence behavior.

There is congruency between aspects of King's (1981) theory and the Health Belief Model (Rosenstock, 1966). Subjectiveness of perceptions is an element of both King's (1981) and the Health Belief Model's (Rosenstock, 1966) definitions. The influence of environment on perceptions is noted in both King's (1981) theory and the Health Belief Model (Rosenstock, 1966). The Health Belief Model (Rosenstock, 1966) proposes that one's environment influences these perceptions. King's (1981) interpersonal and social systems compose the environment for the personal system of the individual. Both King's (1981) theory and the Health Belief Model (Rosenstock, 1966) note the influence of a perceptual process. According to King (1981), behavior is influenced by transactions based on perceptions. The Health Belief Model (Rosenstock, 1966) proposes that a decision-making process weighing perceptions of benefits and barriers influences behavior.

Growth and Development

Growth and development are noted to influence perceptions and are a characteristic of the personal system (King, 1981). Growth and development are defined as changes in the individual based on heredity and environment (King, 1981). Growth and development of the adolescent are known for changes in psychosocial and cognitive functioning.

In terms of psychosocial functioning, adolescence is seen as a transitional period between childhood and adulthood when adolescents are establishing independence from parents (Blos, 1979; Erikson, 1968). During this transitional period, adolescents assume more independence and self-responsibility while reducing dependence on parents and relying more on peers. Therefore, adolescents' interpersonal systems, in relation to parents and peers, are important and may be reflected in perceptions that adolescents have.

In addition to changes in psychosocial functioning, changes occur in cognitive functioning. According to Piaget (1972), the adolescent is capable of abstraction or reasoning in terms of symbols beyond immediate experiences of seeing, hearing, and touching. Piaget's theory of cognitive development can be extended by information-processing system theory (Flavell, 1985). Becoming an expert problem solver in a certain domain depends on knowledge and experience (Chi & Glaser, 1980; Langley & Simon, 1981; Newell & Rosenbloom, 1981). The importance of experiences to cognitive functioning in information-processing theory is congruent with Piaget's theory in that it is noted that the same level of cognitive functioning may not be present for all domains of functioning influenced by one's experiences (Piaget, 1972). Because one's experiences are subjective, one's information and processing of that information are noted to be subjectively influenced (Nisbett & Ross, 1980).

Adolescent development may influence health behavior. Adolescents may be considered inexperienced problem solvers in health areas depending on their knowledge and experience. Being inexperienced problem solvers, adolescents may not consider the consequences of their health behavior; they may not perceive the benefits and barriers to the health behavior.

There is also congruency between aspects of King's (1981) theory and developmental theories. Subjectiveness is an element of King's (1981) definition of perceptions and is noted in information-processing theory in that one's information is subjective. The influence of environment is noted in King's (1981) theory and developmental theory. Perceptions of the personal system are influenced through the socialization process with the family, an interpersonal system, and the socialization the family is influenced by cultural and societal norms of the social system (King, 1983). This is congruent with developmental theory in that relationships with parents and peers are noted to be important for adolescents and especially for socialization of adolescents (Hartup, 1983). Perceptual processes are part of King's (1981) theory in that transactions involve negotiation and exchange of perceptions. These processes are part of information-processing theory in that cognitive functioning is subjectively influenced.

Summary

King's (1981) theory of goal attainment, augmented by the Health Belief Model (Rosenstock, 1966), may be used to promote healthy behavior among adolescents. In transactions between the nurses and adolescent clients, adolescent clients' consideration of perceived benefits and barriers of health behavior may be facilitated. With consideration of perceived benefits and barriers of health behavior, perceived barriers could be anticipated. These perceived barriers could be diminished with plans to handle anticipated barriers, and health behavior or goal attainment could be enhanced.

Cognitive developmental theory supports the need for transactions between nurses and adolescent clients. Adolescents, being inexperienced problem solvers, may not consider the perceived benefits and barriers of health behavior.

King's (1981) concept of transaction is supported by the concept of influential communication, as delineated by Kasch (1986), Kasch and Knutson (1985), and Kasch and Lisnek (1984). Behavioral change occurs through transactions or influential communication, which involves perceptions.

Congruency between aspects of King's (1981) theory, the Health Belief Model (Rosenstock, 1966), and developmental theories exists. Congruency exists in terms of (a) the subjectiveness of perceptions, (b) the influence of one's world of experience on perceptions, and (c) the influence of perceptual processes on behavior. Congruency also exists between King's theory (1981) and influential communication (Kasch, 1986; Kasch & Knutson, 1985; Kasch & Lisnek, 1984). Both King's (1981) concept of transactions and influential communication propose a perceptual process to influence behavior.

Differences in level of abstraction, purpose, and worldview of the theories exist between King's (1981) theory, the Health Belief Model (Rosenstock, 1966), and developmental theory. The concepts of King's (1981) theory are at an abstract level. The concepts of Health Belief Model (Rosenstock, 1966) and cognitive developmental theory are more specific and can be deduced from King's (1981) concepts. The Health Belief Model (Rosenstock, 1966) and information-processing theory are able only to explain and predict behavior based on perceptions or subjectively influenced cognitions. King's (1981) theory of goal attainment provides for prescription (how the nurse and client are to interact, related to perceptions) to change behavior. The world-view of King's (1981) theory is considered to be organismic in that the person is an active participant and holism is assumed (Fawcett, 1989). Cognitive developmental theory also assumes that the person is an active participant and that psychological functioning involves complexly interwoven processes (such as thinking, perceiving, remembering, and feeling) that are more than their summation (Flavell, 1985). In contrast, the Health Belief Model (Rosenstock, 1966) has linear, reductionistic elements.

Testing of King's
Theory of Goal Attainment

Based on King's (1981) theory of goal attainment, a study was conducted to test the effect of a nurse-client transaction on female adolescents' oral contraceptive adherence (Hanna, 1993). King's (1981) perceptions were augmented by perceived benefits and barriers of the Health Belief Model (Rosenstock, 1966) and were specific to oral contraceptives. Based on cognitive developmental theory, the study assumed that female adolescents are inexperienced problem solvers in the area of oral contraceptives. The reader is referred to Hanna (1993) for delineation of the study.

Proposition and Hypothesis

King (1981) proposes that goals are achieved through transactions. The following proposition was tested: "If a nurse and client make transactions, goals will be attained" (p. 149).

For the study, the proposition was deduced to the specifics of female adolescents' oral contraceptive perceptions and adherence. Transactions were specific to female adolescents' perceived benefits and barriers of oral contraceptives, and the goal to be achieved was oral contraceptive adherence. The following hypothesis was tested:

Female adolescent clients who experience the nurse-client transaction regarding perceived oral contraceptive benefits and barriers will have greater oral contraceptive adherence than female adolescent clients who do not experience the nurse-client transaction regarding perceived oral contraceptive benefits and barriers.

Operationalizing the Nurse-Client Transaction

Nurse-client transaction consists of the elements of action, reaction, disturbance, mutual goal setting, explorations of means to achieve goal, and agreement on means to achieve goals (King, 1981). Based on these elements, this nurse-client transaction involved the nurse and adolescent client (a) identifying perceived contraceptive benefits and barriers (action, reaction, and disturbance), (b) confirming the goal of preventing pregnancy by using oral contraceptives (mutual goal setting), and (c) developing a contraceptive adherence regimen to manage perceived contraceptive barriers (agreement on means to achieve goal). The transaction was facilitated by using cards, with each card having a statement that was a potential oral contraceptive benefit or barrier.

The perceptions in the transaction were based on the findings of a preliminary study by the author and perceptions identified by Eisen, Zellman, and McAlister (1985) and Eisen (1988). Examples of perceived benefits were (a) avoidance of pregnancy, (b) wish not to be a mother now, (c) ability to finish high school or go to college, (d) being responsible, and (e) safety and effectiveness of oral contraceptives. Examples of perceived barriers were (a) difficulties around transportation to the clinic, (b) difficulties obtaining birth control pills, (c) difficulties taking birth control pills at the same time every day, (d) difficulties making and keeping clinic appointments, (e) privacy concerns, and (f) birth control being against one's beliefs. The reader is referred to Hanna (1991) for further delineation of the protocol.

Empirical Support for King's Theory of Goal Attainment

The hypothesis was tested with a sample of 51 female adolescents (16, 17, and 18 years of age) who were seeking oral contraceptives. The participants were randomly assigned to either a control or an experimental group. Both groups experienced the clinics' teaching protocol. The experimental group experienced the nurse-client transaction. At the 3-month follow-up, both groups were assessed for oral contraceptive adherence. Analysis of variance was performed to determine if there was a difference in oral contraceptive adherence between the two groups. The .05 level of significance was used. The hypothesis was supported: Female adolescent clients who experienced the nurse-client transaction had significantly greater levels of oral contraceptive adherence than female adolescent clients who did not experience the nurse-client transaction $(F = 4.15, p < .05)$. King's (1981) proposition that goals are achieved through transactions was supported by the findings of the study.

Conclusion

Support is suggested for King's (1981) theory of goal attainment as an intervention or prescription for influencing adolescents' health behavior of oral contraceptive adherence. Female adolescents who experienced a nurse-client transaction around oral contraceptive perceptions had greater levels of adherence than female adolescents who had not experienced a nurse-client transaction around oral contraceptive perceptions. Because female adolescents are inexperienced oral contraceptive problem solvers, the transaction to facilitate consideration of perceived benefits and barriers of oral contraceptives was relevant.

King's (1981) theory of goal attainment has the potential to promote other health behaviors among adolescents. Transactions between the nurses and adolescent clients have the potential for influencing adolescents' perceptions. Nurse-adolescent client transactions around perceived benefits and barriers of other health behavior could influence the health behavior.

King's (1981) theory of goal attainment may be supported by influential communication (Kasch, 1986; Kasch & Knutson, 1985; Kasch & Lisnek, 1984) and augmented by the Health Belief Model (Rosenstock, 1966) and cognitive developmental theory. Congruency between aspects of King's (1981) theory, the Health Belief Model (Rosenstock, 1966), and developmental theories exist. Congruency exists in terms of the subjectiveness of perceptions, the influence of experience on perceptions, and the influence of a perceptual process on behavior. In addition, congruency exists between King's (1981) theory and influential communication (Kasch, 1986; Kasch & Knutson, 1985; Kasch & Lisnek, 1984). Both transactions and influential communication propose perceptual processes between nurses and clients that influence behavior.

References

Baumrind, D. (1987). A developmental perspective on adolescent risk taking in contemporary America. *New Directions for Child Development, 37,* 93-125.

Becker, M. (1976). Sociobehavioral determinants of compliance. In D. Sackett & R. Haynes (Eds.), *Compliance with therapeutic regimens* (pp. 40-50). Baltimore: The John Hopkins University Press.

Blos, P. (1979). The second individuation process of adolescence. In P. Blos (Ed.), *The adolescent passage* (pp. 141-170). New York: International Universities Press.

Chi, M., & Glaser, R. (1980). The measurement of expertise: Analysis of the development of knowledge and skills as a basis for assessing achievement. In E. L. Baker & E. S. Quellmatz (Eds.), *Educational testing and evaluation: Design, analyses, and policy* (pp. 37-47). Beverly Hills, CA: Sage.

Eisen, M. (1988). [Contraceptive health belief scale]. Unpublished scale.

Eisen, M., Zellman, G., & McAlister, A. (1985). A health belief model approach to adolescents' fertility control: Some pilot program findings. *Health Education Quarterly, 12,* 185-210.

Erikson, E. (1968). *Identity: Youth and crisis.* New York: Norton.

Fawcett, J. (1989). *Analysis and evaluation of conceptual models of nursing.* Philadelphia: F. A. Davis.

Flavell, J. (1985). *Cognitive development.* Englewood Cliffs, NJ: Prentice Hall.

Hanna, K. (1991). Effect of nurse-client transaction on female adolescents' contraceptive perceptions and adherence. (Doctoral dissertation, University of Pittsburgh, 1990). *Dissertations Abstracts International, 51,* 3323B.

Hanna, K. (1993). Effect of nurse-client transaction on female adolescents' oral contraceptive adherence. *Image: Journal of Nursing Scholarship, 25,* 285-290.

Hartup, W. (1983). Peer relations. In P. Mussen (Ed.), *Handbook of child psychology: Vol. 4. Socialization, personality and social development* (pp. 103-196). New York: John Wiley.

Haynes, R. (1976). A critical review of the determinants of patient compliance with therapeutic regimens. In D. Sackett & R. Haynes (Eds.), *Compliance with therapeutic regimens* (pp. 26-39). Baltimore: The John Hopkins University Press.

Janz, N., & Becker, M. (1984). The health belief model: A decade later. *Health Education Quarterly, 11*(1), 1-47.

Kasch, C. (1986). Toward a theory of nursing action: Skills and competency in nurse-patient interaction. *Nursing Research, 35,* 226-230.

Kasch, C., & Knutson, K. (1985). Patient compliance and interpersonal style: Implications for practice and research. *Nurse Practitioner, 10*(3), 52-56.

Kasch, C., & Lisnek, P. (1984). The role of strategic communication in nursing theory and research. *Advances in Nursing Science, 7*(1), 56-71.

King, I. (1981). *A theory of nursing: Systems, concepts, process.* New York: John Wiley.

King, I. (1983). King's theory of nursing. In I. Clements & F. Roberts (Eds.), *Family health: A theoretical approach to nursing care* (pp. 177-188). New York: John Wiley.

Langley, P., & Simon, H. (1981). The central role of learning in cognition. In J. R. Anderson (Ed.), *Cognitive skills and their acquisition* (pp. 361-380). Hillsdale, NJ: Lawrence Erlbaum.

Mikhail, B. (1981). The health belief model: A review and critical evaluation of the model, research, and practice. *Advances in Nursing Science, 4*(1), 65-82.

Millstein, S. (1989). Adolescent health: Challenges for behavioral scientists. *American Psychologist, 44,* 837-842.

Newell, A., & Rosenbloom, P. (1981). Mechanisms of skill acquisition and the law of practice. In J. R. Anderson (Ed.), *Cognitive skills and their acquisition* (pp. 1-56). Hillsdale, NJ: Lawrence Erlbaum.

Nisbett, R., & Ross, L. (1980). *Human inference: Strategies and short-comings of social judgment.* Englewood Cliffs, NJ: Prentice Hall.

Piaget, J. (1972). Intellectual evolution from adolescence to adulthood. *Human Development, 15,* 1-12.

Redeker, N. (1988). Health beliefs and adherence in chronic illness. *Image: Journal of Nursing Scholarship, 20,* 31-35.

Rosenstock, I. (1966). Why people use health sources. *Milbank Memorial Fund Quarterly, 44,* 94-124.

·•·—— **19** ——·•·

Analyzing Nurse-Patient Interactions in Japan

TOMOMI KAMEOKA

King's (1968) article titled "A Conceptual Frame of Reference for Nursing" was translated and presented in the *Japanese Journal of Nursing Research* in 1970 (Kobayashi, 1970). It was the first time that King's work was introduced in Japan. In 1976, the book *Toward a Theory of Nursing: General Concepts of Human Behavior*, written by King (1971), was translated and published (Sugimori, 1976). Many Japanese nurses came to know King because of the book (Funashima, 1990). In 1985, King's (1981) book *A Theory for Nursing: Systems, Concepts, Process* was also translated and published in Japan (Sugimori, 1985). King's systems framework and theory of goal attainment were appraised as very useful because many Japanese nurses traditionally set nursing goals (Matsuki, 1986). However, it was said that much

Editors' and Author's Note: The editors and author thank SeonAe Yeo, PhD, RN, University of Michigan School of Nursing, for preparing Table 19.1 in Japanese and providing the English translation.

time would be needed to apply a specific theoretical framework to the real nursing situation in Japan (Funashima, 1990). To date, there are very few reports or studies about application of King's framework and theory in nursing practice, education, or research in Japan.

Some nursing researchers in Japan have questions about nursing practice. Suzuki (1991) conducted research to find the answer to her question as to whether there was a gap between patient needs and the nursing care provided to the patient. She found that clinical nurses had performed many nursing activities, but clinical nurses could not resolve their nursing problems adequately.

In 1992, I conducted a master's thesis about clinical nurses' activities (Kusaka, 1992) with the same question as Suzuki's (1991). As a result, this research further developed Suzuki's findings by doing a theoretical sampling of grounded-theory approach (Glaser & Strauss, 1967). Through the research process, other questions arose. For example, were there situations in which nursing did not result in goal attainment? If so, could specific factors that might have interfered with goal attainment be identified? This latter question led to analysis of nurse-patient interactions to identify what happens in actual nurse-patient situations (Kameoka & Sugimori, 1992; Kusaka, 1991). King's theory of goal attainment was used as a basis for analysis because transaction, a concept within the theory, provides a measure of effectiveness of nursing care (King, 1981, p. 8). In this article, I review nurse-patient interactions from our previous studies in which transactions did not seem to occur. The purpose is to explore the specific factors that interfered with transactions. Knowledge about factors that interfere with transactions could then be used as a teaching tool to maximize nursing care. Throughout this article, I use the phrase "nurse-patient interaction" rather than King's (1981) phrase "nurse-client interaction" because the subjects were hospitalized.

Method

In the theory of goal attainment, King (1981) identified a classification system of nurse-patient interactions. These included the following six elements of interactions: action, reaction, disturbance, mutual goal setting, exploration of means to achieve goal, agreement on means to achieve goal, and transaction-goal attainment (King, 1981, p. 156). This classification system was used as the criterion to analyze nurse-patient interactions in our studies (Kameoka & Sugimori, 1992; Kusaka, 1991).

The collection of data was by nonparticipant observation techniques on two orthopedic wards at two Japanese hospitals. This was done by accompanying nurses on the wards and making detailed notes of nurse-patient interactions. Notes were transcribed to a process recording that included patient's activity, nurse's activity, and an interpretation of the situation. In all, 19 process recordings were reexamined. Specific factors were analyzed and common themes identified. The factors that might have interfered with nurse-patient interactions leading to transactions were found to cluster around the following three themes: (a) differences of perception and inadequate communication between nurse and patient, (b) one-sided (nurse-directed) nurse-patient relationships, and (c) lack of the nurse's concern for the patient and lack of special knowledge of nursing. Cases demonstrating these themes are presented and discussed.

Findings

Theme 1: Differences of Perceptions and Inadequate Communication Between Nurse and Patient

According to the theory of goal attainment, nurse-patient interaction is a process of perception and communication between nurse and patient (King, 1981, p. 145). Accurate perceptions and adequate communication between the nurse and patient facilitate goal attainment (King, 1981, p. 156). However, there were situations that showed differences in perceptions and inadequate communication between nurse and patient.

For example, there was a patient who was on a dietary cure for obesity (see Table 19.1). She had been tested for diabetes and had great concern. She asked a nurse, "I have an acute urge to drink tea recently. So is there a problem?" She was anxious about having diabetes. The nurse answered, "No problem, as tea has no calories;

TABLE 19.1 Process Recording With English Translation

看護婦の言動 Nurse	患者の言動 Client	観察者の視点 Observer
" いかがですか？" "How are you?"	" はい、別にかわりありません。あの、お茶を余り飲まないようにしてみたんだけれど、やっぱり喉が渇くわね。つい飲んでしまうの。大丈夫かしら。糖尿病とかあったらいろいろ検査してるし、わかるんでしょうね。"	変わりないといったん答えたが、気掛かりなことについて尋ねている。飲水制限は、この患者にとって必要なことではないが、なぜか患者は飲水制限をしようとしている。口渇があるので糖尿病ではないかと心配している。
	"..... Nothing has changed. Well, I try not to drink tea as much as I could. But I know I'm thirsty. Can't stop drinking..... Is it OK? If I am diabetic, I should know, because I had many tests, right?"	The client once said that nothing has changed, then she asked about her concern. Though, this client is not restricted for fluid intake, somehow, the client tries to restrict her fluid intake. The client is concerned if diabetes causes her thristy.
" お茶は飲んでも言いですよ。お茶を飲んでふとることはないから。大丈夫ですよ。"		患者はお茶で太るかどうかを尋ねているのではない。患者の質問に答えていない。
"You may drink tea. You won't become fat with tea. It's all right."		The client did not ask if tea could cause obesity. The nurse did not answer the client's question.

it wouldn't make you gain weight at all." The patient said, "I see" and did not ask the nurse any more questions.

Clearly, the patient was worried about the relationship between diabetes and drinking large quantities of liquid. The nurse, however, seemed to assume that the patient was worried about whether or not she would gain weight and answered a different question. Each of them had a different perception of the situation. It could have happened that the nurse understood the patient's concern about diabetes. If so, the nurse's perception would have been similar to that of the patient's and the question would have been answered differently. Now, the question follows as to whether or not the nurse's communication with the patient was adequate in addressing the patient's concern accurately. It seems it was not. It might also have facilitated congruence of perceptions had the patient continued efforts to clarify her concerns to the nurse. In the Japanese culture, patients do not actively express anxiety or concern. However, nurses have a responsibility to maintain open communication (King, 1981, p. 79) and verify perceptions with patients to mutually set goals to be achieved. The importance of accurate perception and adequate communication between nurse and patient in attaining goals was reconfirmed in this case.

Theme 2: One-Sided Nurse-Patient Relationship

According to King's (1981) schematic diagram of the theory of goal attainment, the nurse and patient were drawn as the same size ellipses. This suggests that, although a nurse's role and a patient's role are different, they have the same equality (Funashima, 1989, see esp. pp. 233-253). However, some interactions reviewed for this chapter showed that the patient did not always share an equal relationship with the nurse. This inequality of power is referred to as a one-sided nurse-patient relationship. As a result of inequality of power, decision making is nurse directed.

For example, there was a patient who had had an operative procedure on the cervical spine. Although he was not to move his neck, he was about to move it anyway. The nurse warned him not to move his neck, but she did not explain why she spoke as she did or the goal to be attained by maintaining his position. However, the situation recurred when the patient nearly moved his neck a second time, despite the nurse's warning.

This patient had to keep his neck in the same position for 6 weeks. It is easy to imagine that such a situation would exert heavy stress on him, both physically and mentally. It might have been possible to decrease his stress and make him more comfortable, even if he could not move his neck, if he understood and accepted the goal to be attained. Or perhaps other means for keeping the patient's neck in the same position might have been explored mutually. If the nurse had not directed the patient but, rather, communicated with him, it would have increased his role and power in setting and working toward goals. It does not matter that the directions the nurse provided to the patient were reasonable. Mutual goal setting, exploration of means for goal attainment, and agreement on the means to achieve the goal are less likely to succeed if the nurse directs the patient.

In the history of medical treatment in Japan, the doctor-patient relationship has traditionally been one-sided. Doctors have a tendency to cut off patients' input. This tendency was stronger in Japan than in Europe and the United States (Nakagawa, 1992). The doctor had absolute power in directing care, and the patient had to comply. Discussion of the medical situation with a cancer patient or provision of information for informed consent in medical treatment has only recently gained ground. It seems that the nurse-patient relationship has been strongly influenced by the characteristics of the doctor-patient relationship. However, there is an increasing trend for nurses to question patient care situations. Despite culturally defined customs of deferring to those in higher authority, nurse-patient interactions and practicing one-sided activities by ignoring a patient's wishes are two different things. The theory of goal attainment (King, 1981) is clearly based on involving and respecting patients' active roles in setting and attaining health-oriented goals.

Theme 3: Lack of Nurse's Concern for Patient and Lack of Special Knowledge of Nursing

The focus for nursing is human beings (King, 1981, p. 13). To give patients adequate nursing care, the nurse needs special knowledge. However, interactions in some nursing situations demonstrated a lack of nurses' concern for the patient and a lack of their special nursing knowledge as a basis for care.

An example is as follows: A patient stated to a nurse, "I have a low-back pain, and I'd like to have some compresses." The nurse was just making a nursing record. She then explained the lengthy procedure required to give compresses to the patient without enough assessment. As soon as she had finished explaining it to the patient, she began to write again. Here, the nurse did not demonstrate any activities that could be interpreted as attempts to assess the patient's concerns further or explore other ways to provide pain relief until she could provide the compresses.

In this case, the goal for the patient should have been to allay her pain, and the means for achieving the goal might have been the use of some compresses. But the nurse was not attentive to the patient's problem. Had the nurse showed concern for the patient's problem, used assessment skills and knowledge about pain relief and management, sincerely cared about the patient's pain, and mutually set and validated the goal of reducing pain, the goal of pain relief would have been facilitated. Furthermore, it would have permitted exploration as to whether or not the use of a compress was an appropriate means of achieving the goal and facilitated agreement between the nurse and the patient on the means to achieve the goal.

Following the situation just described, the patient interacted with another nurse. In the latter interaction, all elements of the classification system of nurse-patient interactions were identified. The mutual goal set in that interaction was to allay the patient's pain. The means to achieve the goal were explored, and both agreed to warm the lower back with a hot towel. As a result, the patient's pain was allayed and the goal was attained.

Many situations showed that nurses reacted to questions asked or desires expressed verbally by patients but did not always react to patient problems or concerns that were not expressed verbally. The theory of goal attainment (King, 1981) clearly identifies that communication is nonverbal as well as verbal. According to the theory of goal attainment, the identification of a problem, concern, or disturbance in the patient's environment leads nurse-patient interactions to transactions. When nurses do not have concern from the bottom of their hearts and react only to phenomena that appear on the surface, a patient's actual problems and concern might never be identified. These factors may contribute to nurse-patient interactions that do not lead to transactions. The fact that nurses do not always show concern for patients suggests that nurses might not acknowledge the worth of their nursing profession. Exploration of nurses' sense of value for nursing is an important theme for nursing research and education.

This next case illustrates how the lack of the nurse's special knowledge for nursing might interfere with transactions. A patient recovering from surgery on her hip joint and her nurse set a mutual goal for the patient to be able to walk. In this case, they explored means and agreed to means to achieve the goal. However, the means that they explored and agreed on were inadequate. Despite the patient's ineffective method for strengthening muscle power, the nurse approved of it. If the nurse had had accurate knowledge of rehabilitation, nurse and patient would have selected adequate means, and as a result, interactions would lead to transactions. This suggests that the curriculum of both basic nursing education and continuing nursing education is very important.

Improving Transactions in Nursing

In this chapter, many factors that did not lead to transactions were identified by reviewing nurse-patient interactions at two Japanese hospitals. These cases were analyzed by using King's (1981) classification system of nurse-patient interactions that lead to transactions. According to King, if these elements are present, goals will be attained. Attainment of goals indicates effective nursing care. It follows that if goals are not met, it should be possible to identify the lack of essential elements.

Three major themes were identified: (a) difference of perceptions and inadequate communication between nurse and patient, (b) one-sided nurse-patient relationship, and (c) lack of nurse's concern for the patient and lack of special knowledge of nursing necessary to provide nursing care. In particular, here, the second theme needs further comment because this study has been conducted in Japan. Transactions did not occur in nurse-patient interactions that were characterized by a one-sided nurse-patient relationship. This may be due to the traditional nature of the doctor-patient and the nurse-patient relationship in Japanese culture. However, a theory with a different cultural perspective, if applied to a new culture, could yield a fresh view for nursing practice. Although there are cultural differ-a fresh view for nursing practice. Although there are cultural differences in the nurse-patient relationship, it remains important that the patient participate in setting and achieving goals. It is critical that cultural differences in practice be discussed when deviation from theory is found in theory-testing research.

King's (1981) theory of goal attainment is a normative theory that provides basic knowledge of nursing as a process of interactions leading to transactions in nursing situations. When a nursing situation deviates from a normative theory, factors that contribute to the situation have to be explored. It is important to discover what happens in nurse-patient interactions in which transactions do not occur. It is also important to examine the detailed process by which mutual goals are set, the means to attain the goals are explored, and the means to achieve goals are agreed on in nurse-patient interactions in order to identify what variables facilitate that process. I also believe it is necessary to further develop components of the classification system of nurse-patient interactions in the theory of goal attainment (King, 1981) to answer fully the aforementioned questions about nursing practice. This information will provide useful and concrete means to improve nursing care.

References

Funashima, N. (1989). *Imogene M. King inquirers for current nursing.* Tokyo: Japanese Nursing Association Publishing Company.

Funashima, N. (1990). King's goal attainment theory. *Knago MOOK, 35,* 56-62.

Glaser, B. G., & Strauss, A. L. (1967). *The discovery of grounded theory: Strategies for qualitative research.* Chicago: Aldine de Gruyter.

Kameoka, T., & Sugimori, M. (1992). Application to the King's goal attainment theory in Japanese clinical setting: Part 2 [Abstract]. In *Proceedings of the First International Nursing Research Conference* (pp. 13-14). (Available from First International Nursing Research Conference Secretariat, Tokyo 1992, c/o Japanese Red Cross College of Nursing, 4-1-3 Hiroo Shibuya-ku, Tokyo 150 Japan; phone 81-3-3406-5807; fax 81-3-3406-5849)

King, I. (1968). A conceptual frame of reference for nursing. *Nursing Research, 17,* 27-31.

King, I. (1971). *Toward a theory of nursing: General concepts of human behavior.* New York: John Wiley.

King, I. (1981). *A theory for nursing: Systems, concepts, process.* New York: John Wiley.

Kobayashi, F. (Trans.). (1970). A conceptual frame of reference for nursing [Translated from Imogene King, "A Conceptual Frame of Reference for Nursing," in *Nursing Research, 17,* 27-31]. *Japanese Journal of Nursing Research, 3*(3), 199-204. (Original work published 1968)

Kusaka, T. (1991). Application to the King's goal attainment theory in Japanese clinical settings. *Journal of Japan Academy of Nursing Education, 1*(1), 30-31.

Kusaka, T. (1992). *Clinical nurse's activity for postoperative convalescent patient focused on nursing problem.* Unpublished master's thesis, Chiba University, Chiba, Japan.

Matsuki, M. (1986). A book review: King's nursing theory. *Japanese Journal of Nursing Education, 27*(3), 204.

Nakagawa, Y. (1992). Relationship between a patient and a doctor. *Medical Humanity, 6*(2), 27-31.

Sugimori, M. (Trans.). (1976). Toward a theory of nursing: General concepts of human behavior [Translated from Imogene King, *Toward a Theory of Nursing: General Concepts of Human Behavior*]. Tokyo: Igaku-Shoin. (Original work published 1971)

Sugimori, M. (Trans.). (1985). *A theory for nursing: Systems, concepts, process* [Translated from Imogene King, *A Theory for Nursing: Systems, Concepts, Process*]. Tokyo: Igaku-Shoin. (Original work published 1981)

Suzuki, S. (1991). *Nursing care analysis in clinical nursing activity—focused on nursing problems.* Unpublished master's thesis, Chiba University, Chiba, Japan.

20

Goal Attainment in Short-Term Group Psychotherapy Settings

Clinical Implications for Practice

JOYCE K. LABEN

LARRY D. SNEED

SANDRA L. SEIDEL

With the ever increasing emphasis on providing cost-effective mental health services in the least restrictive environment, providers are challenged to create new and innovative methods for short-term care to consumers. Resources are growing more finite, but the need to provide mental health care continues to grow. Therefore, an interactive systems approach focusing on goal attainment as developed by King (1981) is an ideal theoretical basis for conducting short-term group psychotherapy.

The purpose of the group psychotherapy interventions discussed in this chapter is to describe methods that enable clients to achieve optimum levels of functioning and independence in the community environment. Mutual goal setting between the therapist and the individual, or group members, is achieved via transactions and negotiations based on client values and desires. Goal setting is guided by "objective assessment of functional abilities and disabilities," which provides for "the purposeful planning of goal-directed activities" (King, 1981, p. 8).

King (1981) delineates the fundamental needs of clients as (a) health information in a timely manner when the individual is capable of applying it, (b) preventive care, and (c) assistance for those persons unable to care for themselves. "Health is defined as dynamic life experiences of a human being, which implies continuous adjustment of stressors in the internal and external environment through optimum use of one's resources to achieve maximum potential for daily living" (King, 1981, p. 5). Clients participating in the groups within the community setting require intervention when circumstances interfere with, and inhibit, activities of daily living and independent functioning. The objective of the group projects was to provide participants with information that would help them to identify stressors and develop coping mechanisms and to encourage clients to try out new behaviors.

King's (1981) framework consists of three interacting systems: individuals, groups, and society. The first of the interacting systems is described as the personal systems interacting with the environment through space, time, perception, and self, with growth and development and body image issues taken into account.

Personal System

Space

King (1981) describes space as universal and situational. Individuals have different expectations about space depending on the environment. Areas of privacy gain importance when there is a perception of personal ownership around a given territory.

Three of the groups to be described were conducted in a halfway house. Territoriality was a very important issue because not much space was allotted to each individual. Privacy was nonexistent. The self-esteem group (composed of women) was conducted in a primary care and mental health clinic located in a housing project in an isolated part of town consisting of high-rise apartments and a series of two-bedroom duplexes that fit closely together. The crime rate is high, and people live in fear of their neighbors. Types of crimes vary from family brawls in the common areas to frequent drug trafficking, armed robbery, and murder.

Time

Time is described by King (1981) as being irreversible and universal. Events from the past affect perceptions of the present as well as current and future behaviors, especially if there are major unresolved issues.

The majority of clients who participated in the group psychotherapy projects came from multigenerational families in which histories of violence and emotional, physical, and substance abuse were prevalent. Therefore, a primary focus of the groups was to confront past events to relate historical data to present behavior.

Perception

"Perception is each human being's representation of reality" (King, 1981, p. 20). King describes perception as the relationship of human interaction with the environment, which gives meaning to one's experience of life.

The therapists and other group members had to be able to interpret the perception of each individual and facilitate the cognitive reframing of distortions from past and current life events to assist them in setting helpful goals for changing behavior. Perceptions come from the interactions of sensory organs and the brain processes. Each individual's perception of the world is unique because of past experiences, level of self-esteem, genetic factors, education, and socioeconomic status (King, 1981, p. 20).

Self

The concept of self is made up of personal values and belief systems. It is protected by boundaries governed by the influences of time, space, and perception. Self is related to other persons and to the environment. Self gives one a sense of being unique. The self is goal oriented toward self-fulfillment (King, 1981, p. 27).

Because of crowded living situations in the study populations, there was a lack of physical personal space available. In addition, many of the individuals came from families that were enmeshed, resulting in group members not having a true sense of personal identity. This lack of individuation inhibited group members' ability to develop satisfying and fulfilling interpersonal relationships, particularly with members of the opposite sex.

Growth and Development

According to King (1981, pp. 30-31), growth and development of individuals depend on inherited genetic traits, environmental influences, and interpersonal relationships, which tend to help or hinder an individual's move toward maturity and self-actualization and goal satisfaction. All of the participants in the various groups were at a point in their lives when they were expected to be productively working and caring for family members. It was important to be cognizant of the developmental level of each individual along with the environmental and interpersonal issues, such as abuse, which might inhibit an individual from moving forward toward self-actualization.

Body Image

King (1981) describes body image, an element of the personal system, as being one's view of self, reflected appraisals, and reaction of others to a person's appearance. Personal appearance was very important to members of all of the groups conducted. All members suffered financial deprivation, which gave them fewer resources for purchasing clothing and personal care products.

Interpersonal System

The second interacting system is the interpersonal system, which involves transactions and communication that promotes coping. A person's perceived role and the stress level must be assessed to look at issues in one's life.

Transactions and Communication

The group processes presented illustrate how participants came together to exchange ideas, thoughts, and feelings relative to their individual situations. These interactions encouraged group members to develop behavioral transactions, such as the contemplation of a different approach to solving a family problem. The group leaders and members gave feedback about the proposal, resulting in the identification of new coping mechanisms that facilitated goal setting.

Role

Role places one in a position that requires of an individual certain defined behaviors (King, 1992). Role conflicts come about when the system prohibits one from accomplishing the functions expected of the defined role in society. All group members were in conflict with system-defined roles and their ability to achieve goals defined for that role by society. The prison and halfway house group members had been absent for long periods of time from society, and many of them were at a loss as to how to function when released. Marriages had been severed, their children were older than when group members had been incarcerated, and employment opportunities were minimal. Members of the women's group were faced with serving as heads of the households without the financial resources to carry out the role effectively.

Stress

According to King (1981, p. 95), stress results from physiological, psychological, and social factors. Stress can enhance or inhibit an individual's ability to cope with life's situations. Too much anxiety and stress inhibits a person's ability to function and make appropriate decisions. One's ability to manage stress is affected by how the situation is perceived—that is, as solvable or hopeless. All group members in the various groups had an inordinate amount of internal anxiety that caused them to be unable to cope effectively with financial and emotional problems within their environment.

Social System

The third system, the social system, points to the relationship that individuals have to society and to each other. Social systems are dynamic and must integrate a variety of individual value systems. Power, authority, status, and problem solving are all aspects of whether one is able to function in a social system.

A prevalent theme among participants in the groups centered around feelings of powerlessness and hopelessness. Group members had difficulty perceiving themselves as having authority to make decisions that affect their circumstances. The megasystems of welfare and criminal justice overwhelmed them. When an individual thinks he or she has the system conquered, notification of cancellation of benefits can be perceived as catastrophic. Frequently, group members attributed their feelings of powerlessness to their inability to control both past and present life situations. To overcome this overwhelming sense of hopelessness and to make life-enhancing decisions, a focus on goal setting was established. Group members reviewed various options, including the risks and benefits of the proposed actions. This intervention assisted them in having a sense of power over the system.

Theory of Goal Attainment

When the therapist and the client can agree on the perceptual accuracy of the individual's situation, through mutually defined role expectations, transactions with leaders and other group members can occur, resulting in goal setting, including the steps the client can take to achieve those goals. When role expectations are not mutually defined, role conflict results, which leads to stress. Discussion of performance expectations and the possible outcome of various options to take was completed before final goals were established. Mutual goal setting decreases anxiety and frustration for the individual, especially when the person is able to achieve the desired end.

In the halfway house groups, members were asked to develop life lines to assist them to understand the impact of life events on current behavior and to recognize patterns of behavior that inhibited success in living in the community. In the self-esteem group, all of the members were in individual therapy. However, progress was stalemated. The ability to meet with others in a similar life situation enabled the individuals to interact with each other and to develop goal-setting skills in a nonthreatening environment. Members were asked to identify their stress areas, set goals to alleviate the problem, and compose steps for attainment of those goals.

Self-Esteem Group

Goal-Setting Applications in Therapy Groups

The self-esteem group was conducted at a nurse-managed clinic in an urban housing project. Primary care and psychiatric services are available. Several psychiatrists serve as consultants for prescribing medication, and a social worker is available to handle referrals for social problems, such as referrals to vocational rehabilitation.

Clients came to the clinic both from within the housing project and from the community, generally referred by individuals who had prior contact with the clinic and from private hospitals. Clients were assessed for appropriateness for treatment by the mental health clinical nurse specialists. The typical client evaluated for mental health services is a white female, 41 years of age. More than 60% of the mental health clients are not employed, the mean level of education is the 10th grade, and a majority are on Medicaid. The mean income is below the national average for residents of public housing.

The population in this development is highly mobile, and there is an abiding mistrust and suspicion of neighbors. There have been several violent incidents within the last year, including murders.

From this information, it is not surprising to find that more than 25% of the clients are diagnosed with some form of depression. In the national population, approximately 20% of women have been sexually abused as children (Campbell & Humphries, 1993, p. 34). However, in this mental health clinic population, the figure is 33%. Post-traumatic stress disorder is a prevalent diagnosis, not only from past violent incidents but from more recent recurring events in the community area. Substance abuse issues among the clients were not unusual. Chronic crisis patterns within families were prevalent.

The group consisted of five females. Meetings were held for 1.5 hours, one evening per week, for 10 weeks. The membership was closed after the first meeting. The group membership consisted of all white women with an age range from 29 to 46 years. All of the women had depressive disorders, with one having substance abuse problems and several having been diagnosed with personality disorders. All had a history of some kind of abuse, either emotional, physical, or sexual. Each member was currently seeing an individual therapist in the clinic and had been referred to the group for membership. Each potential member was interviewed prior to joining the group to establish appropriateness for inclusion and to enlist commitment to the group process before the first meeting.

The format of the group was that relaxation exercises were performed at the beginning of each group. This technique enabled the members to center themselves in the group after dealing with their daily crises or stress level. This action assisted members in lowering their anxiety to allow for effective problem solving. The next step was for each member to state how she was feeling physically, emotionally, and spiritually at that moment. After the "go-around," the group entered the planned activity for that session. The group ended with relaxation to prepare them to leave calm and energized.

One objective of the group was to strengthen ego structure through increased self-esteem and sense of self, which might allow the individual to get in touch with feelings, thereby eventually enabling the processing of issues in further therapy. King (1981, p. 31) states that a person moves toward maturity as he or she develops positive

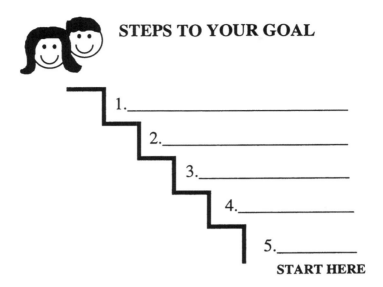

Figure 20.1. Diagram Used to Determine Steps in Meeting a Goal

concepts of self. Another objective was to have each member set an achievable goal for the near future. If the objective could be reached, it would empower the client and give her some sense of control over her life. The members had poor self-images as noted on a pre- and posttest. All of the individuals clearly demonstrated poor self-esteem at the beginning of the group.

The goals set included returning to school, working, moving out of the parents' home, budgeting, controlling finances, and managing enmeshment issues with children. Four of five members achieved their goals.

Each group member was asked to delineate the areas of dissatisfaction in her life and to set a goal related to that area. Steps to goal achievement were reviewed at the third session. A diagram was used to help group members develop steps for meeting the goal (see Figure 20.1). The group members were taught how to examine their perceptions of self through a different visual aid in each session. For example, during one session, the members listed a total of eight of their individual traits, both positive and negative. Each person wrote the traits on wedges of a pie graph developed by the group leader.

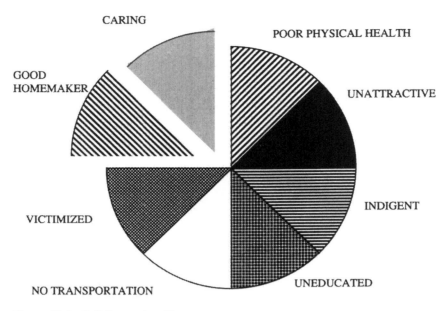

Figure 20.2. Self-Perception Chart

When the pieces of the pie were assembled the client could readily observe how much of herself she viewed as negative (see Figure 20.2). All four members of the group who were present had more designated negative than positive traits. Members of the group tried to assist the individual in exploring the positive traits that were part of the self of each individual. In addition, goals were looked at in relation to the growth and developmental level of each individual client so that goals were not set outside of the developmental reach.

Subsequent group sessions focused on changing some of the negative perceptions of the members and assisting them in recognizing the positive aspects of their personalities. Visual aids were used at every group session. Visual aids reduced cognitive strain in that the members came in already fatigued (Laben, Dodd, & Sneed, 1991, p. 54). Visual aids were also used to reverse negative self-messages by gaining access to the sensory learning centers as well as the cognitive learning centers. Periodically, an assessment was done to establish how far the member had progressed toward attaining the stated goal or goals. At the last group session, each individual

CERTIFICATE

of
Self-Esteem

Awarded to

_____

this 23rd day of November for

achievement of improved

self-worth as noted by her

progress toward the goal of

_____

Signed: _____

Figure 20.3. Certificate of Self-Esteem

received a certificate noting the achievement of her goal (Figure 20.3).
This provided the member with concrete evidence of goal attainment.

Evaluation

In addition to assessment of goal attainment, Yalom's (1985) curative factors were used to measure group progress. Yalom has researched, selected, and measured peer groups through therapeutic elements that operate during a group psychotherapy experience. King (1981, p. 113) writes that development is measured by one's progress within his or her social system, including peer groups. Measurement of the participants' development, through the curative factors described by Yalom, such as installation of hope, was evident during the group process as the members became more verbal and outgoing. They began to have the ability to see themselves in a positive light and to accept positive feedback from both peers and therapists. Physical complaints and statements of hopelessness and helplessness decreased. The curative factor of imparting of information was also present as the various group members shared outcomes of situations with other group members who were going through life ordeals. It was especially helpful when an older member of the group could give feedback to a younger member on how she had managed the same situation successfully or unsuccessfully earlier in life. A third factor of group cohesiveness could also be evaluated as having an impact in that the respect and concern voiced by their peers helped change the group members' prior negative self-perceptions.

Offender Groups

Issues related to group psychotherapy in the treatment of offenders have been well documented in the literature (Bloom, Bradford, & Kofoed, 1988; Nichols, 1984; Ross, Fabiano, & Ewles, 1988; Rule, 1983; Rynerson, 1989). Little, however, has been written concerning the use of nursing theoretical models in the conceptualization and process of group therapy within this population. King's (1981) theory of goal attainment has been the guiding framework applied for psychotherapy with our therapy groups of parolees in a community halfway house.

The halfway house, in which the group therapy projects were conducted, was founded almost 30 years ago and serves both federal and state offenders. It is a private organization governed by a board of directors. Residents are given the opportunity to return to the community on work release. During the several months of their stay, residents can make appropriate plans and arrangements for their lives following release. The majority of residents are nonviolent offenders convicted of their first or second offense. Most are found guilty of crimes such as conspiracy, fraud, theft, and various drug-related offenses.

Three therapy groups have been conducted in this setting. Two groups were led by cotherapists, one male and one female, and one group had three leaders, two women and one man. A total of 20 men (6-7 per group) participated in the project. The length of the group sessions varied from 8 to 12 weeks, with the sessions lasting 1.5 hours. The men's ages ranged from 18 to 63.

Residents in the halfway house are required to maintain employment and pay a portion of their earnings to the house for room and board. Individuals are also required to contribute a percentage of their weekly pay to savings accounts held in their names by the halfway house. Such measures are instituted to promote an environment closely related to life in the community and to assist residents in making the transition from prison to society. Length of stay for residents at the halfway house varies from 30 to 90 days in most cases, although individuals may be allowed to remain in the program for longer periods when additional time is warranted. The house population consists of both men and women. But to date, no female participants have been included in the group project. Several of the men had college degrees, whereas others had not completed high school.

Prior to beginning the group, individuals were interviewed by the therapists for assessment of suitability for the project. Residents were referred by house staff for inclusion in the group. Generally, individuals were accepted if they expressed an interest in the group psychotherapy project and were determined to be cognitively able to function appropriately in a group setting. Additional factors considered in choosing group members included (a) the individual's expression of positive plans following release from the halfway house, (b) a known support system—either family or significant others—in the community, and (c) positive work history with present and past employment.

Laben et al. (1991) presented a framework using the theory of goal attainment (King, 1981) as a method of creating a future-oriented focus for offenders within the community setting. The process involved looking at perceptions of self and tracking growth and development through use of life lines as visual aids to enable the group participants to identify past behavioral patterns that have prevented them from living successfully within the community, and to plan for future goals and attainment of these objectives. Through this process, group members are asked to identify liabilities and assets that can inhibit or enhance the individual's abilities to set and achieve goals. Plans are then created that propose methods of dealing with these issues in a future-oriented perspective. When possible, support from family and significant others is included to provide structure and motivation for participants to maintain the goal orientation.

Recognizing individual personalities and the various psychopathology evident in the group members is an important aspect in attempting positive outcomes within this population. Members of the groups had not been diagnosed with mental illnesses but presented a mixture of psychopathology and personality organization characterized by antisocial features, narcissism, passive-aggressive behaviors, impulsivity, and borderline traits. In addition, individuals in all three of the groups were found to have clinically significant symptomology suggesting affective disturbances. A majority of the men participating in the therapy project also demonstrated poor decision-making abilities and judgment, problems with self-esteem, and difficulty with abstract conceptualizations.

Through the use of visual aids in the form of life lines (see Figure 20.4), past destructive behaviors were approached in a concrete manner that facilitated insight and provided individuals with an opportunity to begin the process of goal formulization and orientation. Confrontation and discussion of decision making were more readily accepted because of feedback of the perceptions of other group members, bringing to light long histories of poor socialization and judgment skills in these individuals. These interventions proved to be useful and necessary for the establishment of goal setting. Clients

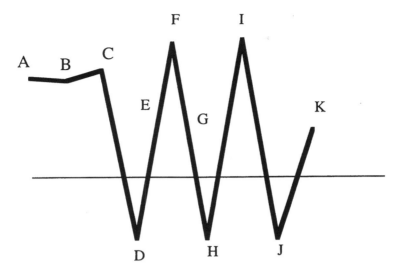

A. Attended grammar school. B. Mother remarried. C. Joined Boy Scouts. D. Breaking and entering, vandalism. E. Doing well in school. F. Part-time job. G. Quit school, 11th grade. H. Dealing drugs, probation. I. Kept job for 1 year. J. Arrested for dealing drugs, 18 months prison. K. Halfway house.

Liabilities	*Assets*	*Plan*
1. Education	1. Personality	1. Obtaining GED
2. Convicted of felony	2. Work history	2. Live with mother and
3. Poor role model	3. Caring	grandmother
for siblings	4. Intelligent	3. Continue in present job
4. No direction in life	5. Savings account	4. After completion of GED,
	6. Supportive family	go to college

Figure 20.4. Life Line Example

were able to identify needed changes in behavior due to an increase in self-knowledge and decision-making skills. Because no follow-up is available after discharge, long-term evaluation of attainment of goals was not possible with this group.

Evaluation

The group members exhibited Yalom's (1985) curative factor of altruism (concern for others) as the weeks went by. Even though the members lived side by side in the house, prior to coming to group, most of them barely spoke to each other. The leaders demonstrated caring to the members by always asking where an absent member was and expressing congratulations and reinforcement if a member had a recent accomplishment. With this modeling and the impact of the groups' allowing members to learn about each other, they began assisting and supporting each other outside the group. Several members helped another from the group solve a perplexing problem in the repair of a car, showing a level of interaction not previously present.

Installation of hope was also a major factor for this group. Those members who had committed white-collar crimes never envisioned a possible criminal sanction for their behavior. Returning to the community was approached with some apprehension as to how former friends and business associates would treat them once released. Finding that the majority of the group members had the same fears enabled them to feel not alone and buoyed by the support of the group that they could start their lives over.

The curative factor of interpersonal learning took place when the various members looked back at their life lines and began assessing the positives and negatives in their lives. With the input and support of other group members, they were able to establish measurable goals, isolating the various steps to those goals. King (1981) states that communication between individuals leads to development of new information, which leads to better decision making. They were able to admit responsibility for past behaviors and make plans for the future, hoping to avoid past mistakes that led to prison terms.

Summary

Persons participating in the groups appeared to benefit when a framework of goal attainment was used (King, 1981). All of the group members had a number of problems in their lives and expressed the themes of helplessness and hopelessness. By employing strategies to look at self-perception, how one transacts with others in their social systems, and using visual aids, the group members could set goals and strive to accomplish them instead of spending most of the group sessions lamenting their life situations. When goals could not be accomplished during the time period for the offender groups, the members could look back at their lives with the life lines and begin planning some positive steps toward the beginning of a crime-free life.

References

Bloom, J. D., Bradford, J. M., & Kofoed, L. (1988). An overview of psychiatric treatment approaches to three offender groups. *Hospital and Community Psychiatry, 39*(2), 151-158.

Campbell, J., & Humphries, J. C. (1993). *Nursing care of survivors of violence.* St. Louis, MO: C. V. Mosby.

King, I. (1981). *A theory of nursing: Systems, concepts, process.* New York: John Wiley.

King, I. (1992). King's theory of goal attainment. *Nursing Science Quarterly, 5*(1), 19-26.

Laben, J., Dodd, D., & Sneed, L. (1991). King's theory of goal attainment applied in group therapy for inpatient juvenile sexual offenders, maximum security state offenders, and community parolees, using visual aids. *Issues in Mental Health Nursing, 12,* 51-64.

Nichols, J. T. (1984). Exorcising the violence of the past. *Delaware Lawyer, 3*(1), 42-44.

Ross, R. R., Fabiano, E. A., & Ewles, C. D. (1988). Reasoning and rehabilitation. *International Journal of Offender Therapy and Comparative Criminology, 32*(1), 29-35.

Rule, W. R. (1983). Exploring paradoxes of happiness in offender therapy. *International Journal of Offender Therapy and Comparative Criminology, 27,* 119-125.

Rynerson, B. C. (1989). Cops and counselors. *Journal of Psychosocial Nursing, 27*(2), 12-17.

Yalom, I. (1985). *The theory and practice of group psychotherapy.* New York: Basic Books.

21

Focusing on King's Theory and Systems Framework in Education by Using an Experiential Learning Model

A Challenge to Improve the Quality of Nursing Care

LISELOTTE ROOKE

In this chapter, a review is presented of the value that Swedish nurses place on conceptual nursing models and theories at different levels of abstraction. The review will use King's (1981) theory of goal attainment and her systems framework as examples. This study focuses on four concepts from King's framework. One aim is to share nurses' everyday experiences in clarifying and interpreting the content of those four concepts and the implications they have for nursing practice. An additional aim is to describe the experiential learning model's role in nurses' learning about conceptual nursing models, thereby decreasing the gap between "theory and practice." These purposes can be seen as a challenge to improve the quality of nursing care.

Progress of Conceptual
Nursing Models in Sweden

An educational reform in Sweden led to nursing education's becoming a part of higher education (Svensk Författningssamling [SFS], 1977). This called for changes within nursing education and nursing practice and also enriched nursing research in Sweden. In 1982, there was a change in policy regarding health care due to the reform of the Health Care Act (SFS, 1982). The reform stressed caring for the individual and that caring would be based on the integrity and autonomy of the individual. Furthermore, good relationships between the patient and the health care staff were emphasized. Both the changes in education and in health care led to an increasing interest in, and a need to develop, the nursing discipline. When a discipline extends, there is an urgent need to develop conceptual models and theories at different levels of abstraction. When this need became obvious in Sweden, it was natural to look beyond the national boundaries and turn to the United States.

In 1982, the new Swedish national curriculum for nursing education stated that nursing conceptual models should be an integral part of nursing education. In basic nursing education, students read about different nursing conceptual models developed by nursing theorists in the United States. Common literature, for example, is Marriner-Tomey's (1989) *Nursing Theorists and Their Work*. Some Swedish textbooks on nursing conceptual models from the United States (Egidius & Norberg, 1983; Rooke, 1991) are also used in nursing education.

Because of the educational reform, nursing conceptual models have been a source of confusion and frustration for nursing educators and nurses. In fact, nurses do not always see if, and how, nursing conceptual models can improve practice. It must be stressed, however, that many nursing educators have shown a great interest in using conceptual nursing models to develop nursing education.

The interest in nursing conceptual models in Sweden is a result of the previously mentioned educational reform, which brought nursing education into higher education. It can be compared with the theoretical development of the nursing discipline in the United States that began in the 1950s. From this time perspective, Sweden is about 20 years behind. However, the gap may not be as big because Swedish nurses and nursing researchers have benefited from the advantages and disadvantages identified in the theory development process in the United States. Thus Swedish nursing educators have had the opportunity to teach *nursing* conceptual models and not, as Meleis (1985) states, to teach about theories of education and administration as was done during the first stages of theory development in the United States.

During the first stage of theory development in Sweden, just as in the United States, there was skepticism among practitioners in nursing regarding conceptual nursing models. Many nurses joined what Meleis (1985) called the "ivory tower" debate. For example, Swedish nurses have asked, "Why make something as simple as nursing so difficult?" Other frequently heard questions were, "Why should we use nursing models from the United States?" and "Why don't we make our own Swedish nursing models?"

In the 1990s, however, a change has been seen. Nurses in practice now show a growing interest in nursing conceptual models, and some nurses see them as useful tools. One example of this interest is the foundation in 1991 of a society called the National Society for Using Nursing Theory in Practice, Education and Research. Today, in 1995, the society has about 300 members—nurses, nursing educators, and nursing researchers.

King's Theory of Goal Attainment

The Swedish Health Care Act (SFS, 1982) states that health care shall build on respect for the patient's right to autonomy and integrity. When Swedish nurses read King's (1981) theory of goal attainment, it is easy for them to accept and integrate King's idea of mutual goal setting between the nurse and the patient. They can easily agree on these specific assumptions from King's (1981) theory:

- Individuals have a right to participate in decisions that influence their life, their health, and community services.
- Health professionals have a responsibility to share information that helps individuals make informed decisions about their health care. (p. 143)

In Sweden, there is an emphasis on implementing individual care planning based on the nursing process. In 1990, the National Board of Health and Welfare set guidelines for nursing practice (Socialstyrelsen Författningssamling [SOSFS], 1990). The guidelines stress that the main task for nurses is setting goals for nursing care and that this shall be done in a dialogue with the patient. Swedish nurses often have a philosophical perspective that respects the patients' autonomy and integrity. One example of this perspective is the involvement of patients in deciding the goals for nursing care, even if goals cannot always be carried out in nursing practice.

King's Systems Framework

The framework consists of three systems: the personal, the interpersonal, and the social (King, 1981). In each system, there are five or six interrelated concepts that have implications for nursing practice. In 1986, King added the concept of learning to the personal system.

King's (1981) framework often inspires Swedish nurses more than the theory of goal attainment. The nurses see the theory of goal attainment as a natural part of their work that does not have to be explicitly discussed. However, the concepts in the personal and interpersonal systems give nurses new ideas to describe and interpret their nursing practice. The concepts provide a new language to describe some parts of their everyday work.

A Pedagogical Base for Learning to Use Conceptual Models of Nursing in Practice

The pedagogical base used in the courses on conceptual nursing models is based on Kolb's (1974) experiential learning cycle. Kolb states that experience plays an important role in learning. According to Kolb (1974; Kolb & Fry, 1975), the experiential learning process consists of four phases: concrete experience, reflective observation, use of abstract concepts, and testing abstract concepts in a new situation. Together, these phases represent two dimensions—namely, the concrete-abstract and the reflective-active.

In the courses, the experiential learning model was implemented by asking the nurses to relate or write a concrete situation (a critical incident) from their own experience (Phase 1). Kolb (1974) states that experience alone does not automatically lead to learning. The individual must be able to observe and reflect on those experiences. In telling a story, there is often a spontaneous moment of reflection. In the reflective phase, both feeling and cognition are involved. Following Kolb's model, the nurses were asked to relate their nursing situations to each other (Phase 2). After relating the situation, they analyzed it by using specific concepts or conceptual models of nursing (Phase 3). In this case, concepts in King's (1981) framework were used. According to Kolb (1974), this process will lead to acting with more consciousness in new situations. As a result, nurses act more skillfully in their everyday work by using theoretical concepts to interpret different patient care situations (Phase 4).

Kolb (1984) points to the similarities between the experiential learning process and the processes of decision making and problem solving. This statement led to the opportunity to connect the learning circle to the nursing process and the steps of assessing, planning, implementing, and evaluating as shown in Figure 21.1.

The nurse has to assess the patient's problems from the patient's reality and concrete experiences. The next two steps, planning and implementing, can be connected to both the reflective phase and Phase 3, using abstract concepts as the focus (reflective observation and abstract conceptualization). By using abstract concepts or conceptual orientations, such as King's (1981) framework, the nurse plans the care together with the patient, implements the care, and evaluates what they have decided and fulfilled mutually (active experimentation). Clearly, the phases are integrated with each other. This is an example of how a conceptual model can guide the nursing

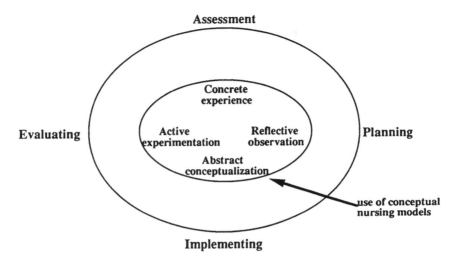

Figure 21.1. The Relationship Between the Nursing Process and Kolb's Experiential Learning Model

SOURCE: Adapted from "Learning and Problem Solving: On Management and the Learning Process," by D. A. Kolb, 1974, in D. A. Kolb, I. M. Rubin, and J. M. McIntyre (Eds.), *Organizational Psychology* (2nd ed., pp. 27-42). Copyright © 1974 by Prentice Hall. Adapted by permission from the publisher.

process. It is my experience that King's framework provides specific and useful concepts that can easily be connected to both the experiential learning process and the nursing process. Using the nursing process *without* any theoretical connection will easily lead to an empty shell. From this point of view, use of a pedagogical method facilitates integration of conceptual models with the nursing process.

Focusing on King's Theory of Goal Attainment and the Systems Framework

I have taught courses for nurses on nursing conceptual models. For examination purposes, the nurses described their interpretation of nursing conceptual models; King's theory of goal attainment and systems framework are often chosen.

Method

The nurses in the previously mentioned courses on nursing conceptual models were asked to describe nursing situations in narrative form. If the systems framework is valid, the situations should have content related to King's concepts. The study was inspired by the tradition outlined by Benner (1984). According to Benner, it is important to uncover the knowledge in nursing practice by describing, in a narrative way, informal nursing knowledge generated from practice. The critical incident method, developed by Flanagan (1949, 1954), provides a rich description of the investigated phenomena by letting nurses relate nursing situations that they have experienced in practice.

Swedish Nurses' Interpretations of Four Concepts in King's Systems Framework

King (1981) writes that the major concepts in her theory of goal attainment are interaction, perception, communication, transaction, self, role, stress, growth and development, time, and space. These concepts are from the personal and interpersonal system. In this study, four of these concepts were investigated: transaction, interaction, perception, and time.

The Concept of Transaction

According to King (1981), transaction is a process of interactions in which human beings communicate with each other to achieve valued goals. This means that the nurse and the patient act mutually to set valued goals. When transactions are achieved, goals are attained, stress is reduced, and satisfaction occurs.

How is the concept of transactions described and interpreted by Swedish nurses? One nurse, who was working with cancer patients, identified that King's (1981) concept of transaction was important regarding these patients. This group of patients frequently have treatments with aggressive chemotherapy. The patients are often well-informed and motivated for their treatments. Both the patient and the nurse must have clearly stated goals, which are set mutually, because they face the side effects and complications together (such as nausea and vomiting, food aversion, loss of hair, tiredness, infections, and bleeding). The main goal is remission of the cancer, and it is essential to work together to attain the goal. To reach transaction, the nurse and the patient need to have confidence in each other and communicate in an appropriate manner. The nurse believed that these types of nursing activities are in accordance with the concept of transaction.

King (1981) states that to reach mutual goal setting, the nurse and the patient ought to have a shared frame of reference such as "facts, beliefs, expectancies and preferences" (p. 82). The related situation can be seen as an example of this statement. Sharing a frame of reference indicates that the nurse must take time to share with the patient. Hence there is a relationship between the concepts of transaction and time.

According to King (1981) an important question is, "What are the essential variables in nurse-patient interactions that result in transactions?" (p. 151). The following variables, based on the related situation and the everyday experience of the nurse, may provide an answer:

- Cancer treatments take a long time, which gives opportunities to develop a deeper relationship between the nurse and patient dyad and to share facts, beliefs, expectancies, and preferences. Time, therefore, might be a valued variable in order to achieve transactions.
- Cancer is life threatening. Individuals in such situations often open up to deeper relationships. Existential individual experiences, therefore, may be an important variable for mutual goal setting between the patient and the nurse.

The Concept of Interaction

King (1981) defines interaction "as a process of perception and communication between person and environment and between person and person, represented by verbal and nonverbal behaviors that are goal directed" (p. 145). The following situation illustrates how this concept has been interpreted by Swedish nurses. It is related by a nurse who also works with cancer patients:

> In the beginning of the treatment, before the patient becomes worse due to the side effects, we work much on getting to know each other. It is important to know how the patient will be treated and how I shall interpret his signals in the right way when he later has difficulties in communicating. It is important to know what he likes, what interests he has, because I must know what is attractive for him when he comes into the phase of passivity. Here, the interaction between the nurse and the patient is crucial.

This example shows that interaction is necessary if the nurse is to be able to assess, plan, implement, and evaluate the nursing care for the patient. The interaction helped the nurse and the patient to clarify the anticipated problems that could develop in the future.

From this nursing example and the nurse's everyday experience, two essential variables for the concept of interaction can be seen:

- *Time.* Nurses must give priority to spending time to get to know the patient.
- *Existential experiences.* The patient knows what the future treatment involves, and he or she also may feel a threat against his or her life. This type of experience affects the interaction between the nurse and the patient, a fact that nurses must recognize.

The Concept of Perception

Perception, the initial phase of the interactive process, is essential in reaching transaction. King (1981) defines perception as "a process of organizing, interpreting, and transforming information from sense data and memory. It is a process of human transactions with environment. It gives meaning to one's experience, represents one's image of reality, and influences one's behavior" (p. 24).

Swedish nurses often state that the concept of perception in King's (1981) framework is difficult to describe and illustrate using a nursing situation. The interpretation does not reflect a lack of value placed on the concept or a lack of their knowledge and experience with perception. Rather, it may be related to the difficulty in finding a nursing situation in which the concept of perception is best represented.

The following nursing situation related by a nursing educator is an example of perception of a patient's situation. The nursing educator described the following:

> I see a well-built man, lying on his right side. He has only the sheet on. The blanket lies at the foot of the bed. Over his left ear he has a dressing. I can see that he is gripping the bed with his left hand. I walk up to the bed and bend over the patient and ask if he wants any help. He does not answer. I repeat my question in a louder voice. The man in the bed lies quite still and says, "I need to go to the toilet." "Can you sit up?" I ask. He does not answer but begins to turn his position in order to lie on his back. Then I see that the man is pale and is sweating. I take my right hand and try to stop the man from changing his position and ask if he does not feel well. "Yes, I am so dizzy. Everything goes round," he answers.

This nursing situation is an example of accurate perception in a situation. The nursing educator's skill in perceiving the patient's condition, followed by validation from the patient, led to an accurate assessment and interpretation of the situation and enabled her to help the patient in the correct way. The nursing educator described that she immediately had the feeling that something was wrong with the patient. She listened to her intuition and perceived, perhaps more intensively, what she saw.

Based on the above situation, an important variable for the concept of perception may be *intuition*. Intuition is defined here as cues that are nearly invisible but can be seen by nurses who have the capacity to perceive these cues' characteristics. Here, the nurse combined what she observed intuitively and the visible signs ("pale and is sweating"). The relationship between perception and intuition is clarified in the next situation, which was related by a midwife:

> As fast as I entered the room, I got a feeling something was wrong. The woman in the bed answered curtly when I asked her something. She looked sad and had something in her eyes that I did not recognize from other pregnant women. She had her hands on

the bed, not on her stomach, as most women do in order to feel the baby. Intuitively, I felt that something was wrong. Before I was going to listen to the heart rate of the child, I asked her if the baby was moving as it had before. Tears came into her eyes and she began to cry. She said that she had not felt the baby move for three days; "The baby is not alive." Her intuition was right.

The Concept of Time

According to King (1981), time is subjective and based on the person's unique experience. As a result, time can be defined only by the individual. King states that the value placed on time by an individual reflects how that person values other individuals. King stresses that time often controls everyday life. The next example illustrates implications for nursing care:

This man is coming to me because he wants an appointment for his operation. He seems to suffer from a lot of stress. Then I suggest a time. He takes his filled diary, and I understand there is really no time for an operation. I know that he should not wait too long because he has a tumor on his neck. We try to find a time and we succeed at last. I give the man the information he needs for the operation, but I feel that he does not really listen. Why? Is it his demanding working life, or is he afraid of the operation and the prognosis? Two days later, the man calls and says that he cannot take the time because something has happened at work. We try again to find a time and managed to do this, but in my opinion it is too far in the future.

The example reflects how time controlled the patient's health-related behavior and how the nurse tried to handle the situation in relation to time and the treatment the patient needed. Therefore, one important variable in relation to the concept of time may be *advocacy*. Although time is subjective and can be experienced only by the person, nurses may have the capacity to advocate for the patient to make time for a health-related behavior. An important variable for the concept of time is this:

- Advocacy, as part of nurses' function, may help patients to manage their time in relation to their health situation.

Discussion

The study identifies the implications for nursing practice of four concepts in King's (1988) systems framework: transaction, interaction, perception, and time. King states, "To find meaning in concepts in everyday living, one examines how to use them. An understanding of a concept is demonstrated by one's ability to apply the knowledge in a new situation" (p. 24). The nursing situations in this study illustrate how nurses find meaning in the concepts and implications for nursing practice. Using concepts is a way of generalizing. When nurses understand the meaning of a concept, it enables them to transfer knowledge from one situation to another. The situations related in this study help to clarify the nature of the concepts.

King's framework also provides structure for using the concepts in practice. The situations related to *transaction* and *interaction* point to the practical use of knowledge of these concepts for improving the quality of care for cancer patients. The situation demonstrating the concept of *time* illustrates the affect on patients' health-related behavior. The situation illuminating the concept of *perception* clarifies the close relationship between perception, intuition, and assessment and the need for nurses to pay attention to this less visible aspect of their knowledge to improve the quality of care.

When nurses were asked to describe nursing situations that mirror concepts of King's systems framework, they often chose situations reflecting the concepts of communication, interaction, transaction, space, stress, and time. The concepts of body image, growth and development, perception, and role were not as often identified in the situations related, nor were concepts from social systems. It is not clear why other concepts, especially those from the personal system, were not identified more often. This is especially true of the concept of perception. Bunting (1988) states that perception has been of interest to nurses since the time of Nightingale. She also points out that, often, perception is included in different conceptual models of nursing. King (1981) claims that "it is essential for nurses to have knowledge of perception if they are to assess, interpret and plan for a client" (p. 24) to attain goals. Further investigations are necessary to discover the distinct means of these other concepts for nurses.

The way in which nurses learn to appreciate and see the meanings of concepts from different conceptual nursing models gives concepts a practical dimension. This can be done through using the critical incident method in which nurses describe nursing situations from their own everyday practice. Kolb's learning circle provides a structure for learning from everyday experience and facilitates understanding of conceptual nursing models. It is my experience that it is important in educational situations to move from a connotative understanding to a denotative description of concepts and not vice versa.

The nurses participating in the courses on conceptual nursing models evaluated King's (1981) theory of goal attainment and the systems framework. Their more informal statements provide a glimpse of the position of Swedish nurses on nursing conceptual models and related theories today. One nurse said that King's theory of goal attainment does not correspond to existing nursing practice in Sweden, but King's assumptions about goal attainment *might be* useful for practicing nurses and for nursing research. This statement can be related to the skepticism that sometimes still exists in practice about conceptual nursing models in general and the fact that theoretical values and assumptions are not always implemented in practice. In contrast, another nurse said that she could easily see examples of King's theory of goal attainment among nurses who worked with goal attainment according to the Swedish Health Care Act (SFS, 1977) and the guidelines from the National Board of Health and Welfare (1990). One nurse asked if the persons who had written the Health Care Act had read King's theory of goal attainment before.

As previously mentioned, nurses in practice are sometimes skeptical regarding the use of conceptual nursing models. This must not be considered unusual. If researchers and theorists do not agree on theoretical statements, assumptions, and definitions, such as the differences between a conceptual model and a theory or the method and the purpose of testing a nursing theory (King, 1991; Nolan & Gordon, 1992; Silva & Sorrell, 1992; Whall, 1989), how could practicing nurses appreciate the usefulness of conceptual models and use them as tools in their everyday work? Using Kolb's (1974, 1984) experiential learning model as a pedagogical base, however, provides an opportunity to bridge the gap between theory and practice. If nurses in education learn to use conceptual models based on experiential learning model guidelines, nurses would more easily find that conceptual models can help them describe and interpret patient situations. This may lead nurses to devote more attention to the utility of conceptual models for practice. The concepts in King's (1981) systems framework provide a sense of pragmatism and, at the same time, lend new dimensions to nurses' interpretation of situations in their everyday practice.

A Challenge to Improve Nursing Practice

The nursing discipline is still emerging and will, I hope, continue to do so. If a discipline does not evolve, there is a risk for stagnation in the development of new knowledge. Regarding the nursing discipline, important concepts have been identified and some have been developed within conceptual models. Theories have been derived and tested. This study expands and clarifies the implications for nursing practice of four concepts from King's (1981) systems framework. This process could also be used for other concepts in nursing frameworks.

There still remains the need to disseminate knowledge of the concepts and the benefits of conceptual models to nursing practice. This will strengthen the link between theoretical concepts and nurses' everyday work. This is nursing's challenge.

References

Benner, P. (1984). *From novice to expert. Excellence and power in clinical nursing practice.* Menlo Park, CA: Addison-Wesley.

Bunting, S. (1988). The concept of perception in selected nursing theories. *Nursing Science Quarterly, 1*(4), 168-174.

Egidius, H., & Norberg, A. (1983). *Theories in nursing practice.* Stockholm: Esselte.

Flanagan, J. (1949). Critical requirements: A new approach to employee evaluation. *Personnel Psychology, 2*(4), 419-425.

Flanagan, J. (1954). The critical incident technique. *Psychological Bulletin, 51*(4), 327-358.

King, I. (1981). *A theory for nursing. Systems, concepts, process.* New York: John Wiley.

King, I. (1986). *Curriculum and instruction in nursing: Concepts and process.* Norwalk, CT: Appleton-Century-Crofts.

King, I. (1988). Concepts: Essential elements of theories. *Nursing Science Quarterly, 1*(1), 22-25.

King, I. (1991). Nursing theory 25 years later. *Nursing Science Quarterly, 4*(3), 94-95.

Kolb, D. A. (1974). Learning and problem solving. On management and the learning process. In D. A. Kolb, I. M. Rubin, & J. M. McIntyre (Eds.), *Organizational psychology* (2nd ed., pp. 27-42). Englewood Cliffs, NJ: Prentice Hall.

Kolb, D. A. (1984). *Experiential learning. Experience as the source of learning and development.* Englewood Cliffs, NJ: Prentice Hall.

Kolb, D. A., & Fry, R. (1975). Towards an applied theory of experiential learning. In C. L. Cooper (Ed.), *Theories of group processes* (pp. 33-57). New York: John Wiley.

Marriner-Tomey, A. (1989). *Nursing theorists and their work* (2nd ed.). St. Louis, MO: C. V. Mosby.

Meleis, A. (1985). *Theoretical nursing: Development and progress.* Philadelphia: J. B. Lippincott.

Nolan, M., & Gordon, G. (1992). Mid-range theory building and the nursing theory-practice gap: A respite care case study. *Journal of Advanced Nursing, 17*(2), 217-223.

Rooke, L. (1991). *Nursing: Theoretical structures for nursing practice.* Stockholm: Almqvist & Wiksell.

Silva, M. C., & Sorrell, J. M. (1992). Testing of nursing theory: Critique and philosophical expansion. *Advances in Nursing Science, 14*(4), 12-23.

[National Board of Health and Welfare and Its Statutes] 15. (1990). *General guidelines from the National Board of Health and Welfare regarding nursing care in health care services.* Stockholm: Norstedts Tryckeri.

Svensk Författningssamling [Swedish Statutes] 218. (1977). *The act of higher education.* Stockholm: Utbildningsförlaget.

Svensk Författningssamling [Swedish Statutes] 763. (1982). *The act of health care*. Stockholm: Norstedts Tryckeri.

Whall, A. (1989). Nursing science: The process and the products. In J. J. Fitzpatrick & A. L. Whall (Eds.), *Conceptual models of nursing analysis and application* (2nd ed., pp. 1-14). Norwalk, CT: Appleton & Lange.

22

Implementation of
Theory-Based Nursing Practice

PATRICIA R. MESSMER

In 1985, **nurse educators** at a large urban public teaching hospital in Southwest Florida presented the work of several nursing theorists to nurse managers, clinical specialists, and staff nurses. After the presentations, a decision was made to use King's theory of goal attainment (King, 1981) because philosophical assumptions about nursing care of patients and their families were similar to the nursing philosophy in this hospital. Although the concepts of the theory were familiar to some of the nurses, many lacked the educational background in nursing theory. In May 1989, the director of Nursing Education and Research (NEAR) developed a systematic plan to implement theory-based nursing practice. The decision to implement theory-based practice occurred simultaneously with several other changes, one of which was computerization of the documentation system. The documentation system needed to be designed to identify and record patient outcomes.

To implement these changes, the vice president for patient services (nursing) appointed the Documentation Task Force, with representation from all levels of nursing. Goals were established along with a timetable. The NEAR director, a member of this task force, was asked to present a plan for implementing theory-based nursing practice and to integrate theory-based practice with the other systems, such as focus charting and marker model. This chapter presents the project for implementing King's theory of goal attainment.

The Project

The project took place in a large urban county-supported hospital on the west coast of Florida. The hospital provides acute care for patients from every socioeconomic group and diverse cultural backgrounds. It is the primary provider of indigent health care for the county. The hospital was featured in *Modern Healthcare* in December 1991 and was recognized by President Bush as one of the top 15 transplant centers in the nation for its high volume and success rate of heart and kidney transplants. The hospital excels in several other specialty areas, such as the trauma, cardiac, burn, neuroscience, and rehabilitation centers. The hospital, affiliated with a university, has both medical and nursing students. Learning experiences are also provided for nursing students from associate degree and practical nursing programs. At the time of the project, 45 master's-prepared nurses (33 master's in nursing and 12 master's in other fields), 260 nurses with BSN degrees, 360 nurses with an associate degree in nursing, 57 diploma graduates, and 145 licensed practical nurses, for a total of 867, were employed.

The Beginning

The philosophy of the Patient Services Department was revised to reflect the assumptions about individuals and families and nursing care based on King's theory of goal attainment (King, 1981, 1989). King was requested to serve as a resource person for the project and became a member of the Documentation Task Force. The NEAR director held meetings with the nurse educators and clinical specialists to plan a continuing education program. In addition, the monthly orientation program was changed to include information about King's theory of goal attainment for the newly employed licensed nursing personnel. The continuing education program consisted of a series of 1-hour conferences orienting the staff to the basic concepts in the theory (Byrne & Schreiber, 1989). This information provided knowledge for the nurses about each concept, the characteristics of each concept, and the definition of each concept. At the completion of studying the concepts, case studies were presented by selected nurses, incorporating all the concepts into a plan of care.

The conferences held with the nurses demonstrated the nurses' knowledge of the concepts and provided examples of nursing care using the concepts. One contact hour credit was given for each conference, and there were a total of 12 conferences; thus most of the nurses received 12 contact hour credits for the continuing education program. This continuing education program helped staff nurses understand the theory and apply this knowledge in their daily practice. Providing examples of nursing care in applying knowledge of the concepts made the conferences pertinent and relevant to these nurses.

The Plan

The director of the Hemodialysis (acute and chronic) Unit expressed an interest in conducting a pilot program. One of the dialysis nurses, who was completing a master's in nursing and had taken a theory course taught by King, felt that theory-based nursing practice would improve patient care. The overall plan to implement theory-based practice included a time schedule for each patient care unit in the renal-transplant and medical-surgical divisions from February 1990 through August 1991.

The Pilot Patient Care Unit

The pilot project was conducted over a 6-month period. A conference room adjacent to the patient care units provided the setting for the 1-hour conferences, held each week for 12 weeks. At the first session, an overview of King's theory and the concepts was presented with time for questions and for discussion. Each week two concepts were discussed. This included the definition and characteristics of each concept. The nurses discussed the implications of this knowledge for nursing care of the patients to whom they were giving care that day or on a previous day. Staff nurses were encouraged to select patients whom they perceived as a challenge to care for and to demonstrate how they would integrate the concept knowledge into the care plan for these patients. Application of the knowledge of the concepts indicated their usefulness for nursing practice.

The director, Dr. King, and a clinical specialist reviewed the content at these 1-hour conferences. Teaching strategies included lecture, questions and answers, case presentations, and discussion of the use of the knowledge gained and how nurses applied that knowledge in their patient care. A handout of the content was given to the staff nurses for their use after the conference. Staff nurses demonstrated their ability to integrate knowledge of the concepts into their clinical practice. Knowledge of the concepts from King's theory made a difference as evidenced by positive patient outcomes in 90% of the charts reviewed, from pretheory to posttheory, using Joint Commission Accreditation Hospitals Organization (JCAHO) criteria.

In one particular instance, staff was experiencing great difficulty with a mildly retarded 21-year-old male. The client was becoming belligerent with staff, ripping out his IVs and becoming abusive to the nurses. Consequently, the staff insisted that his mother remain with him during the dialysis treatment. During the session on the concept of time, the primary nurse in charge of him suddenly realized that for this patient the concept of time was different. The client had a watch on his arm, but if the nurses said that they would return in 20 minutes, the client became angry. However, if the nurses indicated that it was 2 p.m. and that they would return at 2:20, the client would look at the watch and calm down. Soon, the mother was able to leave her son's cubicle and the nurse subsequently wrote a plan of care based on the time concept.

The nurses indicated that as a result of the continuing education program, they had increased motivation about coming to work. They had updated their knowledge base and gained satisfaction from using their new knowledge and communication and interpersonal skills. They viewed each patient as a whole person in this chaotic hospital environment. The head nurse and director of the patient units noted the positive changes not only in their approach to patients and families but also in the nurses' communications and interactions with each other, physicians, and allied health care personnel.

The nurses revised their assessment instrument and developed a flow sheet for identifying mutual goals with dialysis patients and their families. The nurses observed that patients and families expressed their satisfaction with the care received. Of the nurses, 85% recognized that mutual goal setting increased outcomes in dialysis patients relative to nutrition and fluid intake. One of the results of the pilot project was the way in which King was accepted as a nurse member of the group discussion. On the course evaluations, it was noted that knowledge of the concepts of her theory and the process of nurse-patient interaction that lead to transaction and goal attainment (outcome) are relevant for nursing practice. More than 50% of the nurses commented, "We did not realize that theory could make such a difference in our nursing care of patients."

The nurses on this unit provided valuable information for completing this implementation plan. For example, they wrote on the evaluation that a 1-hour conference should be conducted on all three tours of duty (day, evening, and night). They suggested that the 1 hour be changed to a half hour so half of the staff could eat lunch at the time of the conference while the other half of the staff maintained patient care. The nurses felt that the conference would have been more productive if the dialysis nurses had basic knowledge of the concept being reviewed prior to the conferences to facilitate discussion.

The pilot project provided valuable information essential to designing and implementing the continuing education program on all patient units in the hospital. Planning for a housewide continuing education program consisted of developing a self-learning module orienting the staff to the basic concepts in the theory, including the definition and characteristics of each concept. The nurses were expected to complete 32 questions related to the concepts as one component of evaluation for the continuing education program. The module was pretested and could be completed in 5 hours, so the nurses were given 5 contact hours of credit for the self-study. Successful completion of the self-study validated the learner's ability to apply King's concepts. The NEAR director and nurse educators reviewed the responses and noted any knowledge deficit. On one occasion, one of the nurses taking the self-study had no basic knowledge of child development. The self-study was revised to include child-adult growth and development with specific examples of the application of the King's theory to the different stages.

Implementation of the Project

Following the pilot test, the trauma unit was designated as the next patient care unit to implement King's theory. Prior to the continuing educational program, the NEAR director mandated that all the nurses successfully complete the self-study module on King's concepts and view a 15-minute film that portrays application of King's concepts (the videotape was produced at Sunnybrook Medical Center, Toronto, Canada).

King, the NEAR director, and nurse educators implemented the continuing education program, which included 1-hour conferences on day, evening, and night shifts. Suggestions from nurses on the pilot unit were incorporated in revising the time schedule for the conference. For example, half of the nurses would attend the first 30-minute conference and half would attend the second 30-minute conference.

This schedule provided adequate time to review two concepts and discuss application of the knowledge of the concepts in daily practice. This also provided adequate coverage for all patients in the trauma unit during the hour designated for the conferences. The conferences were conducted at mealtimes and held twice so that all nursing staff could attend. King was available as a consultant on a periodic basis. The NEAR director and nurse educators were available on a full-time basis.

Evaluation of the Project

Because determining patient outcomes was a priority, measuring those outcomes as a result of implementing theory-based practice became imperative (Byrne-Coker et al., 1990; West, 1991). King's process of interaction that leads to transactions and to goal attainment (outcomes) is an integral element in this outcome-oriented theory. Methodology included measuring patients' satisfaction with nursing care pre- and postimplementation of King's concepts. The sample consisted of 50 patients from the general surgical inpatient pilot unit and 50 patients from two other units not implementing theory-based practice. The 100 patients were surveyed prior to implementation of theory-based practice. Hinshaw and Atwood's (1982) Patient Satisfaction Instrument (PSI), a valid and reliable instrument, was administered to all 100 patients. This instrument (see the appendix) measures patients' attitudes toward nurses and their nursing care.

Nurse educators who were not caregivers on the units conducted the survey. Criteria for participating in the study were the following: (a) must be over 18 years of age, (b) must be at least 3 days postoperative, (c) must have not been on more than one unit since surgery, and (d) must have the ability to read and understand English or Spanish. Another 100 patients were surveyed in September 1992, after the implementation of theory-based practice, to determine if there was a significant difference in the level of patient satisfaction between the pilot unit and the other units. Data were analyzed using SAS (Statistical Analysis Systems).

Results

Initial evaluation of the project consisted of 111 completed surveys for the experimental group and 69 for the control group, with 93 surveys for 1991 and 87 surveys for 1992. The results indicated that the mean age for the experimental group was 49.5 years ($SD = 1.5$), and for the control units, 45.2 years ($SD = 2.0$). There was a different proportion of males in 1992 (70%) for the experimental unit compared to males in 1991 (43%). This also occurred for the males in the control group for 1992 (30%) compared to 1991 (57%). There was no difference in the females in 1992 (70%) compared to 1991 (70%) for the experimental group and no difference in the females in 1992 (30%) compared to 1991 (30%) for the control group. There was an interaction in Item 1—"The nurses should be more attentive than they are." This indicated that the patients became more dissatisfied in the controlled unit ($M = 3.6$, $p < .02$) compared to the experimental group, which did not change from 1991 to 1992.

There also was an interaction in Item 5—"The nurses should be more friendly than they are." The control unit disagreed more in 1992 ($M = 3.2$) than did the experimental group ($M = 3.8$, $p < .04$) and was marginally significantly different from the control units in 1991 ($M = 3.7$, $p < .096$). For Item 19—"The nurses are not just patient enough."—the control unit in 1992 disagreed less ($M = 3.5$) than in 1991 ($M = 4.0$, $p < .026$). Nevertheless, the experimental group disagreed more than the control group in both 1991 and 1992. For Item 25—"The nurses are skillful in assisting the doctor with procedures."—there was no change from 1991 to 1992 for the control group. However, the experimental group agreed more in 1992 ($M = 1.8$) than in 1991 ($M = 2.1$, $p < .068$).

Analysis of variance revealed a significant difference between the level of satisfaction according to gender ($F = 3.92$). When controlling for gender, females reported a higher level of satisfaction for the following items:

Item 1   The nurses should be more attentive than they are ($F = 2.22$).

Item 4   I feel free to ask the nurses questions ($F = 2.45$).

Item 5   The nurses should be more friendly than they are ($F = 2.10$).

Item 15   Nurses give good advice ($F = 3.51$).

Item 19   The nurses are not just patient enough ($F = 2.61$).

Item 25   The nurses are skillful in assisting the doctor with procedures ($F = 3.12$).

Although providing a conceptual basis for nursing care did not significantly improve the level of patient satisfaction in all the questions, there is evidence that the continuing education program did increase the level of awareness and made a difference in certain questions for the females. Perhaps the males are more critical, especially after a surgical experience, when completing a survey instrument. This finding warrants further study on examining the difference between males' and females' perspectives of patient satisfaction. The questions reported to demonstrate a difference are examples of the application of the concepts of goal attainment. These findings indicate that the nurses grasped the concepts to affect patient care positively.

Summary of Implementation
of Theory-Based Nursing Practice

Implementation of the Department of Patient Services' philosophy of nursing based on King's theory of goal attainment required a formal and systematic continuing education program for nurses employed at this institution. A continuing education program was designed for currently employed staff nurses at one hospital to gain knowledge of King's theory of goal attainment concepts. In addition, the continuing education program was incorporated into the orientation of newly employed nurses. The concepts in King's theory provide substantive basic knowledge for using the nursing process of assessing, planning, implementing, and evaluating nursing care.

King's nursing process demonstrates how nurses identify mutual goal setting with patients and their families, explore means to achieve goals, agree on the means, and then move toward goal attainment. This process helps nurses document nursing care and evaluate its effectiveness because patient goals set and attained are recorded and represent patient outcomes (King, 1992). After the implementation of theory-based practice on the trauma unit, a new admission assessment tool incorporating King's concepts was implemented for all the medical-surgical units.

The NEAR director, nurse educators, and clinical specialists coordinated the implementation of this project with the clinical director, head nurse, and staff nurses in each unit. The pilot project provided information that was used to develop a self-learning module related to the concepts in King's (1981) theory of goal attainment. The nurse educators conducted follow-up evaluations in the patient care units at 3-month and 6-month intervals to observe for use of the knowledge gained. The implementation of this continuing education program serves as a model for other hospitals. The results of the project demonstrated that implementing theory-based nursing practice can result in improving the level of patient satisfaction.

Appendix

Patient Satisfaction of Nursing Care Survey	Strongly Agree	Agree	Uncertain	Disagree	Strongly Disagree
1. The nurses should be more attentive than they are.	1	2	3	4	5
2. Too often, the nurses think you can't understand the medical explanation of your illness, so they do not bother to explain.	1	2	3	4	5
3. The nurses are pleasant to be around.	1	2	3	4	5
4. I feel free to ask the nurses questions.	1	2	3	4	5
5. The nurses should be more friendly than they are.	1	2	3	4	5
6. The nurses are people who can understand how I feel.	1	2	3	4	5
7. The nurses explain things in simple language.	1	2	3	4	5
8. The nurses ask a lot of questions, but once they find the answers, they do not seem to do anything.	1	2	3	4	5
9. When I need to talk to someone, I can go to the nurses with my problems.	1	2	3	4	5
10. The nurses are too busy at the desk to spend time talking with me.	1	2	3	4	5
11. I wish the nurses would tell me about the results of my test more than they do.	1	2	3	4	5
12. The nurses make it a point to show me how to carry out the doctor's orders.	1	2	3	4	5
13. The nurses are often too disorganized to appear calm.	1	2	3	4	5
14. The nurses are understanding in listening to my problems.	1	2	3	4	5
15. The nurses give good advice.	1	2	3	4	5
16. The nurses really know what they are talking about.	1	2	3	4	5
17. It is always easy to understand what the nurses are talking about.	1	2	3	4	5
18. The nurses are too slow to do things for me.	1	2	3	4	5
19. The nurses are just not patient enough.	1	2	3	4	5
20. The nurses are not precise in doing their work.	1	2	3	4	5
21. The nurses give directions at just the right speed.	1	2	3	4	5
22. I'm tired of the nurses talking down to me.	1	2	3	4	5
23. Just talking to the nurses makes me feel better.	1	2	3	4	5
24. The nurses always give complete enough explanations of why tests are ordered.	1	2	3	4	5
25. The nurses are skillful in assisting the doctor with procedures.	1	2	3	4	5

References

Byrne, E., & Schreiber, R. (1989). Concept of the month. *Journal of Nursing Administration, 19*(2), 28-32.

Byrne-Coker, E., Fradley, T., Harris, J., Tomarchio, J., Chan, V., & Caron, C. (1990). Implementing nursing diagnosis within the context of King's conceptual framework. *Nursing Diagnosis, 1*(3), 107-114.

Hinshaw, A., & Atwood, J. (1982). A patient satisfaction instrument: Precision by replication. *Nursing Research, 31*(3), 170-175.

King, I. (1981). *A theory for nursing: Systems, concepts, process.* Albany, NY: Delmar.

King, I. (1989). King's systems framework for nursing administration. In B. Henry, C. Arndt, M. Di Vicenti, & A. Marriner-Tomey (Eds.), *Dimensions of nursing administration* (pp. 35-44). Boston: Blackwell.

King, I. (1992). King's theory of goal attainment. *Nursing Science Quarterly, 5*(1), 19-24.

West, P. (1991). Theory implementation: A challenging journey. *Canadian Journal of Nursing Administration, 4*(1), 29-30.

·•·—— **23** ——·•·

Theory of Goal Attainment in the Context of Organizational Structure

MARY LUE JOLLY

CYNTHIA KELSEY WINKER

Several theories exist in the extant body of knowledge in nursing. Current knowledge in management science indicates that the complex nature of health care systems demands a systems approach to practice and management (Kirby, 1991). Marriner-Tomey (1989) identifies four nursing theorists who derive their work from systems theory: Dorothy Johnson, Sr. Callista Roy, Imogene King, and Betty Neuman. This chapter explores the possible implementation of theory-based practice in a hospital nursing service department using King's (1981) theory of goal attainment.

The Need for Theory

Theory generated for theory's sake is not useful to a practice discipline such as nursing. The real purpose of theory in a practice discipline is to serve as a foundation for both practice and research. Theory that can be applied in practice and used to create an environment in which quality patient care can be delivered will benefit the clients served as well as advance the profession of nursing.

In 1981, King, recognizing the need for nurses to understand the complexity of the environment in which they practiced in order to achieve professional and organizational goals wrote, "Above all the nurse is accountable to the person who receives care" (p. 119)—which is to say, the client gives meaning to the practice of nursing. According to King (1989), the nurse functions in several arenas: (a) nurse and client, (b) nurse and nurse, and (c) nurse and physician. However, regardless of the arena, the ultimate focus is the care of the individual. In the past few decades, nursing research, guided by theory, has contributed to the efficacy and continuous improvement of nursing care. Nurse academicians and researchers have found direction for research and curriculum development around various theories. Now, nurse executives in various health care settings are beginning to use theory to guide practice and to shape the culture of the nursing department. The combined influences of management research and literature plus experiences would lead the nurse manager to expect that theory-driven practice will produce five effects: (a) creation of consistency in performance, (b) assurance of constancy of purpose, (c) development of a common ground for problem solving, (d) identification of a means by which to evaluate successes, and (e) provision of a road map for future planning (Deming, 1986; King, 1989; Kirby, 1991; Meleis & Jennings, 1989; Peters & Shaterman, 1982). In this chapter, unless otherwise noted, *client* refers to the manager and the staff members with whom the interaction takes place.

Consistency of Performance

A mutually agreed upon theoretical framework will necessarily reduce variation in practice habits and style, thereby creating more consistent and predictable performance. Both managers and clinicians will be more consistent in their performance if organized around a common framework of thinking. The proper selection and maintenance of a theory for practice will create an environment where expectations are more clear regarding the nurses' performance. Clear expectations will promote harmony and balance between the nurse and the external environment, enabling the nurse to function optimally and to deliver nursing care in a way that will meet and exceed patient expectations (King, 1981).

Constancy of Purpose

Deming (1986) coined the phrase "constancy of purpose," indicating that an organization must know at what it is to be successful as it moves forward into the future. Constancy of purpose strives for improvement of product and service. Integrating theory into a nurse's practice will create, over time, a clear and constant purpose and will shape the parameters of discipline. Peters and Shaterman (1982) write, "Good managers make meanings for people as well as money" (p. 27). The patient provides purpose and meaning to nursing. A nursing theory properly chosen and consistently used in both the delivery of patient care and the management of the environment in which it is delivered will keep the focus of the improvements on the patient.

Common Ground for Problem Solving

When problems are identified, exploration of solutions will occur along conceptual lines present in the theory by which the nursing staff practices. Much as when a researcher frames a research question within a theory, a committee or group of staff members can explore problems encountered within the theory on which their practice is based. Common ground will guide the nursing clinicians and managers more directly to solutions without having to go through unnecessary and time-consuming efforts to bring the group to thinking along the same conceptual and philosophical lines. Meleis and Jennings (1989) suggest that tension between the practitioner and the manager can be reduced when they have a common framework. In addition, theory can guide the nurse executive in problem solving with other departments and outside agencies.

Practice Evaluation

Success can be measured, evaluated, and documented as described in the theory. For example, when nurses use King's (1981) theory, patients who are able to meet their own goals are a documentable success. Similarly, when the nurse manager and the clinical director agree that the manager will pursue a master's degree this, too, can be documented after completion.

Future Planning

Both the successes and failures in implementing theory in practice can assist in future planning. The process can be continuously improvised through the identification of needs and deficits in the ability to fulfill both patients' needs and the needs of the organization. Effective future planning is critical if the organization is to remain viable in an increasingly competitive environment.

Theory Selection

The implementation of theory-based practice, although promising for the future of nursing and patient care, should not be implemented in any setting without thorough analysis and careful selection of the most appropriate and useful theory for the particular setting. Although the need for theory-driven nursing practice is becoming more popular in hospital settings, it is certainly far from the norm. One might speculate that selection of a nursing theory may intimidate nurse executives who, unless they were educated in the past 10 to 12 years with advanced degrees in nursing, may not be familiar with the subject and may be somewhat intimidated by the challenge. At a minimum, nurse managers may not be convinced of the value of theory-based practice and may see its implementation as one more stress in their practice. Meleis and Jennings (1989) suggest that tension between practitioners and managers can be reduced when they share a common framework.

The nurse executive should consider the following components when evaluating which theory is most compatible with the health care organization's mission and most useful to the practitioners:

(a) the nursing department and the larger system in which it functions; (b) the philosophy, mission, and structure of the nursing service organization; (c) the ease of communication of the theory to others outside of nursing; (d) the consistency of the theory with the state of the science and art of both management and nursing practice; and (e) the ability to use the theory in practice, management, and peer relationships (King, 1989).

System Considerations

In considering the nursing system and the larger system in which it operates, the nurse administrator must be conscious of who and what will be affected by the implementation of theory-based practice. These include, but are not limited to, other departments in the organization, physician relations, and resource constraints. Accepting the assumptions of systems theory, one must believe that any change in one part of a system will have an impact on the other parts of the system. Therefore, a change so fundamental and pervasive as theory-based nursing will affect all parts of the hospital. The nurse administrator must be cognizant of this impact and select a theory compatible with not only the nursing division but also the overall system.

Philosophy, Mission, and Structure

The theory must be consistent with the philosophy and mission of the nursing division. Philosophy and mission should not be altered to fit the theory but, rather, the theory should be chosen for its match. Either structural issues, such as methods of charting and management information systems, must be compatible with the theory, or the nurse administrator must be ready to adapt them to fit the theory.

Communication With Others

Selecting a theory with widely understood terminology will facilitate the communication of the theory to both nursing and non-nursing personnel within the system. This will enable understanding and support for theory-based practice in the organization as a whole.

State of the Art and Science in Management and Practice

The theory selected should reflect the most current thinking in both nursing practice and management theories if it is to be successful in the modern competitive health care arena. The theory will have more credibility with both nurses and nonnurses in the system if the concepts are consistent with the most visionary thinking in the industry. In nursing organizations, shared governance and participatory management are becoming the norm. This form requires mutual goal setting at all levels of decision making (Elberson, 1989).

Use Beyond Patient Care

The theory should be applicable to relationships other than patient care. The nurse applying theory in practice should be able to apply the same concepts in any human interaction process. Application of the theory should be effective in all relationships—nurse to nurse, nurse to manager, manager to senior manager, and senior manager to chief executive officer.

King's Theory of Goal Attainment

Imogene King (1971) has conceptualized a framework from which the theory of goal attainment was developed. Initially, she intended her work to be used as a "conceptual frame of reference for nursing . . . to be utilized specifically by students and teachers . . . researchers and practitioners to identify and analyze events in specific nursing situations" (p. ix). According to King, her thinking was heavily influenced by general systems theory, originally conceived by Ludwig Von Bertalanffy (1968) in his work as a biologist, but which evolved to influence the behavioral and management sciences as well (Davidson, 1983). Systems theory has emerged as a way of dealing with changes and managing complex organizations and is a fundamental building block of the current movement in quality management or continuous quality improvement (Kirby, 1991).

Theory serves as a looking glass on the world. Using the theory of goal attainment (King, 1981), one views human beings as total persons interacting with their environment. The total person includes the experiences of individuals in the past, in the current situation, and in the future.

King's (1971, 1981) framework describes three dynamic, interacting systems: personal, interpersonal, and social. Personal systems are represented by each individual as an unique and distinct functioning system. When the individual enters into interaction with another the interpersonal system is created. Interpersonal systems are represented in King's framework as a group of at least two individuals in interaction. The social system is the third system in which both groups and individuals stand as elements in interaction within the immediate environment.

The theory of goal attainment (King, 1981) emanates from the interpersonal system within the framework. The concepts central to the theory are interaction, perception, communication, transaction, role, stress, growth and development, time, and space. The following definitions are paraphrased from King's 1981 text.

Interaction. Human interactions assist the nurse in gathering information. Observation, physical presence, and verification are key elements of interaction. For example, during an interaction, the clinician assesses the readiness of the patient for progress in goal setting and attainment, or the nurse manager assesses the clinician's readiness to pursue a master's degree.

Perception. Perception is the manner in which each individual conceives reality. The perceptions of each person involved in the interaction are critical and can shape the interaction. Factors in the environment such as difference in educational background of nurse as well as sensory changes can influence perceptions. Perceptual congruence between the nurse manager and staff members expedites communication and goal attainment (King, 1989).

Communication. This is the informational process for transmitting messages. Verbal and nonverbal symbols are involved in the communication process. Both the behavior of the patient and the behavior of the nurse are critical in the communication process. This process contributes to perception and interaction.

Transaction. Individuals communicating for the purpose of goal setting and the means to achieve goals composes the process of transaction. Roles, values, expectations, and perceptions of each person contribute to the success of the transaction.

Role. The set of behaviors expected of an individual in a given situation constitutes the definition of role. The outcome of care can be influenced by the perceptions each individual has of the role of the nurse and the role of the patient.

Stress. Stress is a state produced by interactions between the environment and the individual. The environment is both internal and external. The nurse is expected to reduce stressors by providing information and assisting the patient in verbalizing concerns. Giving patients control over their care as appropriate will reduce stress in some situations as well.

King's (1981) theory of goal attainment clearly meets the last three criteria for theory selection mentioned in the preceding section. By design, King's language is simple and nonacademically oriented. Although in some circles she has been criticized for this simplicity, she believes that the ease of communication is essential for nurses and those nonnurses in the context in which nursing is practiced (I. King, personal communication, August 1992).

King advocates the systems approach, which is consistent with forward-thinking leaders in management science. General systems theory has given management science a holistic approach to improve organizational systems and is particularly able to address the complex organization with multiple interacting systems (Kirby, 1991). Health care organizations, of which nursing is an integral part, are clearly one of the most complex suprasystems in today's world. King's (1981) theory offers nursing the opportunity to organize the approach to patient care in a manner consistent with the most recent trends in management science and is compatible with the world of quality management and continuous quality improvement practiced in many health care institutions today.

The propositions of this theory are based on assumptions about humans as open systems in interaction with their environment.

Therefore, the theory is applicable to any human interaction. Nurses who understand and practice King's theory will be able to apply the theory in every human interaction.

The other two criteria recommended for use in theory selection can be addressed only within the organization itself. However, prior to discussing implementation issues, the assumption is made that King's theory is compatible with the nursing and hospital system and consistent with the philosophy, mission, and structure of the nursing organization.

Implementation

According to Smith (1993), any organizational change must consider three dimensions: people, structure, and tasks. In considering people, the nurse executive must consider all individuals and departments this change will affect. The capabilities of the people who will be performing different assignments must be considered as well. The structure of the implementation plan and the organization must be addressed. Finally, the nurse executive must consider if the theory fits the tasks required by all customers of the organization.

The nurse executive considering implementing theory-based practice would be well-advised to conduct some preliminary research of similar organizations that have had experience in the process. This knowledge will better prepare the nurse executive and convince key people of the need and value of the change.

The chief executive officer must be convinced of the value of theory-based practice. King's (1981) theory can be comprehended and implemented more easily than some other nursing theories because of the simple and commonly understood language and its compatibility with current management science. Once agreement in principle has been reached with hospital management, a period of exploration with senior nursing management must be held.

The nurse executive must seek answers to these questions: Is the theory simple? Is it applicable to all interactions? Is it representative of sound management theory as well as patient care management? Is the theory compatible with the philosophy, mission, and structure of the organization? The discussion of the concepts and premises of the theory during the selection process will identify the structural elements that will require support and change.

An implementation team is formed to oversee the necessary changes and tasks involved in implementing theory-based practice. The members selected for the team must be thoroughly conversant with the theory of goal attainment (King, 1981). This team is responsible for developing an implementation plan for the organization. Included in the implementation plan is the selection of a unit to pilot the implementation process as well as the development of a training program. Ideally, the nurse manager and nurse clinicians from a unit will volunteer to be this pilot unit. A training program is written for participant self-study to ensure consistency in the content that is presented. Ongoing training and reinforcement must be consistent and constant. If at all possible, visits by the theorist should be planned during various phases of the implementation process. Important to the sustenance of theory-based practice is the allocation of funds in the budget for maintenance, consultation, and education. Contacts with other users of the theory should be initiated and maintained. A network of users can be valuable in preventing mistakes and providing encouragement in difficult times. Schools of nursing using the theory as a basis for their curricula should be included in the network as a support for ongoing development and research possibilities.

The demonstration of value is critical to the ongoing success of the project. Proctor and Rhodes-Auton (1986) identify three areas affected by theory-based practice: (a) the attainment of cognitive skills contained in the theory; (b) the perceptions of the patient and nurses regarding the nursing care; and (c) the impact of theory-based practice on patient outcomes. Each of these areas must be evaluated to demonstrate the value of theory-based practice not only for the organization but for the discipline of nursing. Plan to tell the story to others through publication in professional journals and in-house communication vehicles.

King has indicated that institutions have attempted to implement theory-based practice using her model but have failed in some cases (I. King, personal communication, August 1992). This failure has resulted because the originator did not ensure perpetuity. Only the individual who started the process was invested in the theory, not the organization. When the individual left the organization, the continued use of the theory disappeared. King believes that to ensure successful implementation and ongoing maintenance, the theory (a) should become an integral part of an orientation program, (b) should not be "owned" by one person in the organization, and (c) should not compete with too many other projects (I. King, personal communication, August 1992).

Summary

In summary, theory-based nursing using King's framework (1981) offers the opportunity for nursing to focus on patients, improve care, and improve professional relationships. Many issues compete for attention in the health care system. However, if the patient is to remain the focus, theory-based nursing must not become one of the trivial efforts on the "to do list" of nurse executives but must become one of the vital few efforts in the strategic planning of forward-thinking, customer-driven health care institutions.

References

Davidson, M. (1983). *Uncommon sense: The life and thought of Ludwig Von Bertalanffy.* Los Angeles: Tarcher.

Deming, W. E. (1986). *Out of the crisis.* Cambridge: Massachusetts Institute of Technology, Center for Advanced Engineering Study.

Elberson, K. (1989). Applying King's model to nursing administration. In B. Henry, C. Arndt, M. Di Vincenti, & A. Marriner-Tomey (Eds.), *Dimensions of nursing administration: Theory, research, education, practice* (pp. 47-53). Boston: Blackwell.

King, I. M. (1971). *Toward a theory for nursing: General concepts of human behavior.* New York: John Wiley.

King, I. M. (1981). *A theory for nursing: Systems, concepts, process.* New York: John Wiley.

King, I. M. (1989). King's systems framework for nursing administration. In B. Henry, C. Arndt, M. Di Vincenti, & A. Marriner-Tomey (Eds.), *Dimen-*

sions of nursing administration: Theory, research, education, practice (pp. 35-53). Boston: Blackwell.

Kirby, K. (1991). Organizational change: The systems approach. In M. J. Stahl & G. M. Bounds (Eds.), *Competing globally through customer value. The management of strategic suprasystems* (pp. 219-252). New York: Quorum.

Marriner-Tomey, A. (1989). *Nursing theorists and their work.* St. Louis, MO: C. V. Mosby.

Meleis, A., & Jennings, B. M. (1989). Theoretical nursing administration: Today's challenges tomorrow's bridges. In B. Henry, C. Arndt, M. Di Vincenti, & A. Marriner-Tomey (Eds.), *Dimensions of nursing administration: Theory, research, education, practice* (pp. 7-18). Boston: Blackwell.

Peters, T. J., & Shaterman, R. H. (1982). *In search of excellence.* Philadelphia: Harper & Row.

Proctor, D. M., & Rhodes-Auton, V. (1986). Documenting care in the medical intensive care unit: Change theory in action. *Critical Care Nurse, 6*(5), 80, 82-86.

Smith, M. C. (1993). The contributions of nursing theory to nursing administration practice. *Image: Journal of Nursing Scholarship, 25*(1), 63-67.

Von Bertalanffy, L. (1968). *General systems theory.* New York: George Braziller.

—— 24 ——

Theory-Based Practice in the Emergency Department

MICHELLE BENEDICT

MAUREEN A. FREY

The standards of practice for the Emergency Nurses Association call for the explicit use of nursing process to ensure high-quality care for patients in the emergency department (ED) (Dains et al., 1991). The nursing process, however, is a generic, four-step problem-solving method. As such, it must be based on, or driven by, theory (Mitchell, 1992). The purpose of this chapter is to demonstrate the use and utility of Imogene King's (1981) theory of goal attainment for organizing and delivering patient care in the ED.

Traditionally, nursing has used theories from many other disciplines, such as sociology, psychology, anthropology, and medicine. More recently, there has been an increased awareness of the need to identify, explicate, and use nursing theories and conceptual frameworks as the basis of practice (Fawcett, 1989; Fitzpatrick & Whall,

1989; Huch, 1988). The systematic structures of the various frameworks provide guidance for assessing, planning, implementing, and evaluating nursing care within a distinct context and format. Communication is enhanced by the use of common terminology, care is more holistic, and, overall, quality of care is improved (Fawcett et al., 1987; Johnson, 1987; Meleis, 1991). In addition, explicit use of a nursing theory or conceptual framework in practice contributes to examination of the validity of the framework or theory in terms of doing what it purports to do (Fawcett, 1989; Fitzpatrick & Whall, 1989; Silva & Sorrell, 1992).

Some of the same factors that make ED nursing exciting also limit the use of nursing process and hinder the delivery of quality care. Emergency nurses are faced with a diverse patient population and various acuity levels. Often, judgments about the acuity of the situation are not shared by the patient and the nurse. Nurse-patient interactions are often brief, intense, and subject to many interruptions. There is a tendency to concentrate on the presenting problem, particularly the medical aspects of the presenting problem, and not on the patient as a whole. A review of the literature indicated no explicit applications of nursing conceptual frameworks or theories to guide nursing in the ED despite the obvious benefits of and need for doing so.

Relevance of King's Framework and Theory to Emergency Department Nursing

King's (1981) systems framework consists of three open interacting systems: Individuals are personal systems, groups of two or more form interpersonal systems, and larger groups with common interests and goals constitute social systems. Systems are interrelated. King identified concepts relevant to understanding each system. Knowledge of the concepts guides nurses in a variety of diverse situations.

King defines nursing within the context of the theory of goal attainment, which is derived from concepts of the personal and interpersonal systems. These concepts are perception, communication, interaction, transaction, self, role, growth and development, time, space, and stress. King states, "Nursing is a process of human interactions between nurse and client whereby each perceives the other and the situation; and through communication, they set goals, explore means and agree on means to achieve goals" (1981, p. 144).

The theory of goal attainment (King, 1981) includes a process of perception, judgment, actions, and reactions by both the nurse and the patient that leads to nurse-patient interactions. During this process, the nurse assesses, observes, interprets, and clarifies, and the patient observes, interprets, asks questions, and gives information. Interactions include mutual goal setting and also lead to transactions. Goal attainment also occurs within transactions. Outcomes of both interactions and goal attainment are measurable.

King proposes that mutual goal setting will lead to goal attainment. Patients who actively participate in goal setting will be more likely to achieve goal attainment. And when goals are attained, health is restored or improved. Health is viewed as the ability to function in social roles.

The nursing process is described as a set of interrelated actions: assessment, planning, implementing, and evaluating. Concepts relevant to the nursing process addressed in the theory of goal attainment (King, 1981) include perception, communication, interaction, decision making, goal setting, transactions, and goal attainment.

The theory of goal attainment (King, 1981) is consistent with the *Standards of Emergency Nursing Practice* (Dains et al., 1991). Standard 6, Component A, "Nursing care is evaluated on a continuous basis to determine progress or lack of progress toward patient outcome and patient goal attainment" (p. 81), provides support for using the theory of goal attainment.

Application of the Theory of Goal Attainment

Figure 24.1 shows modification of the theory of goal attainment for use in the ED. In the ED, a patient's first encounter with a nurse is with either the triage nurse or the treatment nurse, depending on the severity of the presenting problem. Due to this two-step process of assessment, illustrated in Figure 24.1, King's theory may be repetitive or partially repetitive. The following application involves

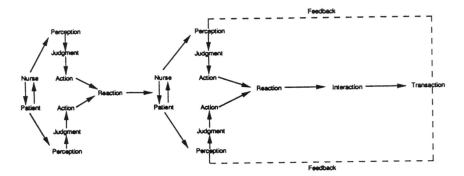

Figure 24.1. Modification of King's Theory of Goal Attainment for Use in the Emergency Department
SOURCE: Adapted from *A Theory for Nursing: Systems, Concepts, Process*, p. 145, by I. King, 1981. Copyright © 1981 by Delmar Publishers. Adapted by permission of the publisher.

a 25-year-old female (Ms. B.) who presented with the chief complaint of arm pain due to a fall. She drove herself to the ED, was ambulatory, and presented alone.

Assessment

At the time of initial encounter, Ms. B. stated to the triage nurse, "I fell and need my arm checked. Nothing else hurts." Information given by the patient provided the nurse with a starting point for assessment. Initial assessment, primarily done by observation, revealed obvious and fairly recent bruising of the left eye, a swollen and bruised lower lip, and swelling distal to the left forearm. In addition, the nurse noted that Ms. B's affect was flat, she had difficulty maintaining eye contact, and she spoke very little, usually only in response to direct questions. The triage nurse's perception and subsequent judgment was that Ms. B's description of the incident was not consistent with the injuries noted. Furthermore, on the basis of her knowledge of battered women, the nurse also suspected that Ms. B was a victim of domestic violence, most likely at the hand of a significant other. Ms. B's presentation in the ED for a non-life-threatening injury was an indication of reaching out for help with a very serious, health-threatening problem (Campbell & Sheridan, 1989). The action taken by the triage nurse was to ask the patient directly if she had been assaulted, to which Ms. B. stated, "Yes." This was immediately followed by the statement, "I do not want to press charges; I only want to have my arm checked."

Use of a structured framework for nursing practice facilitates communication between nursing staff members. When Ms. B was seen by the treatment nurse, the triage nurse was able to report her perception (discrepancy between event and injury), judgment (domestic violence), and action (asking directly about assault) as well as the patient's reaction (affirmation of beating and statement of preferred course of action). During the treatment phase, further physical assessment revealed no additional injuries or visible evidence of abuse. Psychosocial assessment revealed that Ms. B. was married to the man who assaulted her, they had no children, and this was not the first episode of physical injury. In discussing the incident further, Ms. B. stated that she "egged him on," indicating that she assumed responsibility for the assault. She also stated that she "did not need help" and that "the situation will get better." These are not uncommon remarks and attitudes of victims of domestic violence, although research indicates that for most couples, the violence increases in frequency and severity over time (Campbell & Humphries, 1993).

Further communication and interaction were directed toward helping Ms. B. understand that physical assault was never appropriate, regardless of one's behavior. The nurse offered information on resources for women, such as hotlines, shelters, and support groups. The nurse also validated the normalcy of Ms. B.'s responses, pointing out that additional physical symptoms could result from her husband's potential for violence. During this interaction, Ms. B was able and quite willing to verbalize feelings and talk about the incident. This is not always the case, especially when the patient is accompanied to the ED by the abuser, who often acts to isolate the victim (Campbell & Sheridan, 1989).

Plan

In terms of setting goals with Ms. B., it was critical that the goals be mutually set (King, 1981). Although some health professionals might assume that the only goals were to press charges and assist the patient in leaving the abusive situation, the literature does not support this reality (Campbell & Humphries, 1993), especially when the victim sees the incident as a minor event and does not perceive it as ongoing abuse. In this case, the mutually agreed-upon goal was determination of the extent of the injury and pain relief.

The nurse identified an additional goal that influenced the interaction process, primarily that of empowering the patient. This goal of empowerment is based on King's (1981) assumptions about nurse-patient interactions, which state:

- Health professionals have a responsibility to share information that helps individuals make informed decisions about their health care.
- Individuals have a right to participate in decisions that influence their life, their health, and community services.
- Goals of health professionals and goals of recipients of health care may be incongruent.
- Individuals have a right to accept or reject health care. (p. 143)

Implementation. The following plan (means to achieve the goals) was agreed on by the nurse and Ms. B. and implemented: X-rays, pain relief, and ice packs to minimize swelling. In addition, Ms. B. stated that she would think about taking the information offered about shelters and other resources while in the X-ray department.

Evaluation. After returning from the X-ray department, Ms. B stated that she had thought about their conversation and did not want any help at the present time. However, she did request and accepted referral information (pamphlets) "in case I need it later." Because the X-rays did not indicate any fractures, her forearm was wrapped and she was given a prescription for analgesics prior to discharge.

Using a nursing process format, the nurses recorded the interaction on the ED record. Based on the theory of goal attainment (King, 1981), this included documentation of the nurse's perceptions, judgments, objective data, and actions as well as the client's verbal and nonverbal behavior, which indicated her perception, judgment, and actions. The plan of care, which included mutual decision making about goals, exploring the means to attain goals, and agreement on the means to attain goals was implemented within a transaction (the active participation and exchange of values between a nurse and a client). Evaluation of the outcomes of the interaction and transaction in terms of the goals attained completes the documentation of the nursing process.

Documentation of suspected or actual assault, as in this case, is essential. Although Ms. B was not pressing charges at this time, she may choose to do so at some future date. Although battery is a crime in all 50 states, reporting obligations vary, and reporting is usually not required unless the victim presses charges. Fortunately, this is changing in some areas.

Summary

This case study demonstrates the many advantages of using an explicit nursing framework as a basis for nursing practice. First, it provides structure in the form of concepts that are useful in understanding individuals as personal systems, the interactions of personal systems, and how these interactions influence health. A major strength of the framework is its emphasis on perceptions and their influence on behavior, both the nurse's and the patient's. In this case, if the nurse had not used the special knowledge and skill of nursing in making her own assessment, abuse, as the underlying threat to health status, may not have been identified.

The framework also directs the nurse to validate perceptions and judgments. In addition, it actively involves the patient in planning and implementing nursing care, recognizing patient perceptions and needs. Finally, the theory of goal attainment (King, 1981) provides a mechanism for facilitating communication between health professionals, which provides continuity of care. Most important, it provides a nursing framework for implementing the nursing process with the overall objective of improving the health outcome of clients.

References

Campbell, J. C., & Humphries, J. C. (1993). *Nursing care of survivors of family violence.* St. Louis, MO: C. V. Mosby.

Campbell, J. C., & Sheridan, D. J. (1989). Emergency nursing interventions with battered women. *Journal of Emergency Nursing, 15*(1), 12-17.

Dains, J., Alexander, E., Jordan, K., Lyle, N., Schoerger, J., Rice, M., & Ingalls McKay, J. (1991). *Standards of emergency nursing practice* (2nd ed.). St. Louis, MO: C. V. Mosby Year Book.

Fawcett, J. (1989). *Analysis and evaluation of conceptual models of nursing* (2nd ed.). Philadelphia: F. A. Davis.

Fawcett, J., Cariello, F. P., Davis, D. A., Farley, J., Zimmarro, D. M., & Watts, R. J. (1987). Conceptual models of nursing: Application to critical care nursing practice. *Dimensions of Critical Care Nursing, 6*(4), 202-213.

Fitzpatrick, J. J., & Whall, A. L. (1989). *Conceptual models of nursing: Analysis and application.* Norwalk, CT: Appleton & Lange.

Huch, M. H. (1988). Theory based practice: Structuring nursing care. *Nursing Science Quarterly, 1*(1), 6-7.

Johnson, D. E. (1987). Evaluating conceptual models for use in critical care nursing practice. *Dimensions of Critical Care Nursing, 6*(4), 195-197.

King, I. (1981). *A theory for nursing: Systems, concepts, process.* New York: John Wiley.

Meleis, A. (1991). *Theoretical nursing: Development and progress* (2nd ed.). Philadelphia: J. B. Lippincott.

Mitchell, G. J. (1992). Specifying the knowledge base of theory in practice. *Nursing Science Quarterly, 5*(1), 6-7.

Silva, M. C., & Sorrell, J. M. (1992). Testing of nursing theory: Critique and philosophical expansion. *Advances in Nursing Science, 14*(4), 12-23.

PART IV

EVALUATION

State of the Science
and Future Directions

JACQUELINE FAWCETT

ANN L. WHALL

K**ing began to develop** the general systems framework and theory of goal attainment in the 1960s, when nursing was striving for status as a science and hence as a legitimate profession. This book underscores the continuing value of King's work and its impact on the advancement of nursing science and the professional practice of nursing. In fact, the book represents a virtual compendium of the ways in which a conceptual model of nursing and middle-range nursing theories can be used to address a variety of problems within the discipline of nursing.

State of the Science

A major strength of King's work is its clear division into an abstract and general conceptual model, the general systems framework, and a middle-range theory, the theory of goal attainment. King (1989) identified the unique focus of her work as "human beings interacting with their environment" (p. 150) and, more specifically, as "individuals whose interactions in groups within social systems influence behavior within the systems" (p. 152). Particular attention is given to the continuing ability of individuals to meet their basic needs so that they may function in their socially defined roles.

A comprehensive analysis of King's work indicates that she values the client's participation in his or her nursing care as well as valuing the client's right to accept or reject the care offered by nurses and other health care professionals. Moreover, King places equal value on the nurse's and the client's perceptions of any given situation. In fact, her definition of nursing as a process indicates that both nurse and client participate in setting goals and determining the means to achieve the goals (Fawcett, 1995).

King's general systems framework and her theory of goal attainment represent substantial contributions to the discipline of nursing. The concepts and propositions of the framework, together with the content related to each concept of the personal, interpersonal, and social systems, form the conceptual-theoretical systems of nursing knowledge that are needed for various nursing activities. Furthermore, the theory of goal attainment is a major contribution to the growing body of distinctive nursing theory.

The general systems framework provides a comprehensive discussion of the metaparadigm concept of person. Indeed, King's descriptions of the major concepts and subconcepts associated with personal systems, interpersonal systems, and social systems provide more specification of individuals, groups, and society than is usually found in a conceptual model. In addition, King has provided a clear and concise definition of the metaparadigm concept of health. She also defined illness and related that concept to her definition of health by indicating that disturbances in the dynamic state that is health are regarded as illness or disability. Furthermore, King defined and described the metaparadigm concept of nursing in a comprehensive manner and clearly identified the goal of nursing as health.

The utility of the general systems framework and the theory of goal attainment is based on the fact that King (1975) deliberately constructed the framework from "recurring ideas or . . . concepts that were undergoing verification through systematic investigation" (p. 37). Thus the linkage of the theory of goal attainment with the general systems framework represents a conceptual-theoretical system of nursing knowledge that emphasizes nursing care based on empirically adequate scientific findings and enduring traditions deemed acceptable by society.

Some chapters in this book document the utility of the general systems framework for middle-range theory development. Those chapters demonstrate how diverse strategies can be used to develop middle-range theories from King's framework. Sieloff's theory of departmental power is a prototype for theory reformulation (see Chapter 5). Wicks's theory of family health (see Chapter 8), Frey's theory of families, children, and chronic illness (see Chapter 9), and Doornbos's theory of family health in the context of chronic mental illness (see Chapter 15) are prototypes for theory derivation from the general systems framework. Those latter three authors also demonstrate how a conceptual-theoretical system of nursing knowledge can be tested through empirical research. Hobdell's work demonstrates the development and testing of an explicit conceptual-theoretical-empirical structure that links the general systems framework with the two existing middle-range theories of person perception theory and the theory of chronic sorrow and with empirical indicators in the form of valid and reliable paper- and pencil-questionnaires (see Chapter 10).

Other theoretical work has been directed toward the expansion of the concept of health within the context of King's general systems framework. Sieloff presents an expansion of King's definition of the health of personal systems to social systems. Consistent with the origins of King's framework, Sieloff draws heavily from general system theory (see Chapter 11). Winker presents an expansion of King's notion of health that takes into account the general systems theory ideas of transformation and equifinality, as well as the metaphysical principle of teleology (see Chapter 4).

Other chapters in this book, along with previously published reports, document the utility of the general systems framework and theory of goal attainment for nursing research and nursing practice. In fact, evidence supporting the contention that use of the general systems framework and theory of goal attainment leads to improvements in individuals' health status has been accruing for several years. For example, Smith's (1988) case presentation suggested that mutual goal setting resulted in attainment of goals and enhanced client health. Kohler (1988) indicated that mutual goal setting and agreement on means to achieve the goals increased compliance with the medication regimen. DeHowitt (1992) stated that individual psychotherapy guided by the theory of goal attainment increased a male patient's own goal setting and goal attainment, which in turn increased the patient's positive feelings about himself and his feelings of progress in therapy. Furthermore, Martin's (1990) results supported the effectiveness of an intervention on men's awareness of prostate and testicular cancer. In addition, Hanucharurnkul and Vinya-nguag's (1991) results supported the effectiveness of intervention based on the theory of goal attainment on several measures of postoperative recovery.

Additional evidence is presented in several chapters of this book. For example, Fawcett, Vaillancourt, and Watson report a case study demonstrating the value of King's framework in the complex care of a woman suffering from severe side effects of cancer chemotherapy (see Chapter 14). Hanna reports that her study results supported the efficacy of a nursing intervention based on the theory of goal attainment on adolescents' oral contraceptive adherence behavior (see Chapter 18). Using the case study format, Alligood explains how the use of King's framework and theory enhanced the nursing care of a 17-year-old girl who had suffered acute multiple trauma when hit by a car while riding her bicycle and a 40-year-old woman with chronic back pain (see Chapter 16). Laben, Sneed, and Seidel report that group psychotherapy based on the theory of goal attainment had beneficial outcomes for women who participated in a self-esteem group and for parolees in a community halfway house (see Chapter 20).

The utility of the general systems framework and the theory of goal attainment for nursing administration is also documented in this book. For example, Messmer describes the implementation of King's work in a large urban teaching hospital and reported that use of the framework and theory enhanced patient satisfaction with nursing care (see Chapter 22).

Still other chapters in this book, along with other publications, support King's contention that the general systems framework and the theory of goal attainment are applicable cross-culturally. For example, Spratlen (1976) built on King's early work to develop "an approach to nursing education, research and practice which incorporates the cultural dimensions of attitudes and behavior in matters of health" (p. 23). Rooda (1992) described a conceptual model for multicultural nursing that she developed from the theory of goal attainment. She noted that the model provides direction for nursing practice and research and prepares nurses to provide holistic nursing care in a global society. In addition, Rooke, in Chapter 21 of this book, describes the meaning that Swedish nurses ascribed to King's concepts of transaction, interaction, perception, and time. And Kameoka, in Chapter 19, identifies factors that impede transactions in two Japanese hospitals and uses the theory of goal attainment as a structure for suggestions related to enhancing nurse-patient interactions.'

Directions for the Future

Our evaluation of the chapters in this book was guided by Walker and Avant's (1988) caveat that beginning works and works in progress should be subjected to a standard different from that for works that have stood the test of time in the marketplace of ideas. More specifically, Walker and Avant maintain that critical evaluation of new efforts should be tempered with a tolerance for creativity, so that new efforts will be allowed to flourish and grow into formal systems of knowledge.

With Walker and Avant's (1988) caveat in mind, we identified five areas that would benefit from additional thought and study. One area is King's discussion of the metaparadigm concept of environment. In particular, although King (in personal communication to R. Martone, July 25, 1989) notes that her concept of social systems "explains environments and internal [environment] is explained in [the] communication concept," further discussion of the environment would be desirable.

The second area is King's view of wellness and illness. In a 1990 article, King revealed that she has rejected the idea of health as a continuum of wellness to illness because that is a linear notion.

Using the same reasoning, it may be inferred that she also rejects the idea of health as a dichotomy of wellness and illness. That inference, however, requires a response by King to avoid misinterpretation of her conceptualization of wellness and illness.

The third area is the further development of implicit middle-range theories into formal theories. Alligood, Evans, and Wilt explain how the concept of empathy can be viewed within the context of the personal, interpersonal, and social systems of the general systems theory. Their work represents the development of an implicit middle-range theory of empathy (see Chapter 6). Rooke's work is another example of the development of an implicit middle-range theory. Using King's notion of space as a guide, Rooke employed an inductive approach to describe personal space and social space (see Chapter 7). Both of those implicit theories could be transformed into formal middle-range theories by presenting explicit propositions about the relevant concept dimensions and their connections.

The fourth area is the issue of congruence between the general systems framework and middle-range theories that were developed within the context of other frames of reference. Sieloff achieved congruence by carefully reformulating an existing theory into her theory of departmental power (see Chapter 5). Coker and her colleagues systematically examined the nursing diagnoses developed by the North American Nursing Diagnosis Association (NANDA) for their congruence with King's conceptual framework and accepted only those that were relevant to the concepts of the personal, interpersonal, and social systems (see Chapter 13). Similar care must be taken in future attempts to link the general systems framework to existing middle-range theories.

The fifth area is continued empirical testing. The fact that the theory of goal attainment has been tested and found to be empirically adequate is significant. Additional tests of the theory of goal attainment, as well as the other middle-range theories that have been derived from the general systems framework, would add to the evidence regarding the empirical adequacy of the theories and their generalizability across various situations and client populations. Furthermore, the credibility of the general systems framework requires continuous investigation by means of systematic tests of conceptual-theoretical-empirical structures derived from the framework, the theory of goal attainment or other relevant theories, and appropriate empirical indicators.

Conclusion

The chapters of this book add to the growing volume of literature that provides specific and explicit documentation of the utility of the general systems framework and theory of goal attainment for nursing research, education, administration, and practice. The contents of this book should lay to rest, once and for all, the all too frequently heard charge that conceptual models of nursing and nursing theories are mere intellectual musings that have no utility for practical activities (Frissell, 1988; Hayne, 1992; Kenny, 1992). Furthermore, the preceding chapters, along with this chapter, should help all nurses to understand that the intellectual products of a nurse theorist are not accepted as an ideology that cannot be subjected to empirical tests and modified on the basis of those tests. Finally, the contents of this book document the advances in knowledge development and use that can be achieved when creative forces within nursing are supported. We, along with the editors and other contributors, hope that this book will serve as an exemplar for all nurses who are using or would like to use conceptual models of nursing and nursing theories to guide their nursing activities.

References

DeHowitt, M. C. (1992). King's conceptual model and individual psychotherapy. *Perspectives in Psychiatric Care, 28*(4), 11-14.

Fawcett, J. (1995). *Analysis and evaluation of conceptual models of nursing* (3rd ed.). Philadelphia: F. A. Davis.

Frissell, S. (1988). So many models, so much confusion. *Nursing Administration Quarterly, 12*(2), 13-17.

Hanucharurnkul, S., & Vinya-nguag, P. (1991). Effects of promoting patients' participation in self-care on postoperative recovery and satisfaction with care. *Nursing Science Quarterly, 4,* 14-20.

Hayne, Y. (1992). The current status and future significance of nursing as a discipline. *Journal of Advanced Nursing, 17*, 104-107.

Kenny, T. (1992). Nursing models fail in practice. *British Journal of Nursing, 2*, 133-136.

King, I. M. (1975). A process for developing concepts for nursing through research. In P. J. Verhonick (Ed.), *Nursing research* (Vol. 1, pp. 25-43). Boston: Little, Brown.

King, I. M. (1989). King's general systems framework and theory. In J. P. Riehl-Sisca, *Conceptual models for nursing practice* (3rd ed., pp. 149-158). Norwalk, CT: Appleton & Lange.

King, I. M. (1990). Health as the goal for nursing. *Nursing Science Quarterly, 3*, 123-128.

Kohler, P. (1988). Model of shared control. *Journal of Gerontological Nursing, 14*(7), 21-25.

Martin, J. P. (1990). Male cancer awareness: Impact of an employee education program. *Oncology Nursing Forum, 17*, 59-64.

Rooda, L. A. (1992). The development of a conceptual model for multicultural nursing. *Journal of Holistic Nursing, 10*, 337-347.

Smith, M. C. (1988). King's theory in practice. *Nursing Science Quarterly, 1*, 145-146.

Spratlen, L. P. (1976). Introducing ethnic-cultural factors in models of nursing: Some mental health care applications. *Journal of Nursing Education, 15*(2), 23-29.

Walker, L. O., & Avant, K. C. (1988). *Strategies for theory construction in nursing*. Norwalk, CT: Appleton & Lange.

Index

About the Authors

Martha Raile Alligood, Ph.D., R.N., is a Professor in the College of Nursing at the University of Tennessee at Knoxville, where she teaches nursing theory in the graduate programs. Formerly, she chaired the Department of Psychophysiological Nursing and was Associate Professor in the College of Nursing at the University of South Carolina. She held a graduate faculty position at the University of Florida and was Director of the School of Nursing at Ohio University in Athens. She received her doctorate in nursing from New York University, her master's from Ohio State University, and a B.S.N. from the University of Virginia. She has had international nursing experience in Zimbabwe, Africa, where she directed the nursing program at Mashoko Christian Hospital while associated with Central Africa Mission. Her research includes testing theory derived from Rogers's Science of Unitary Human Beings across the adult life span—specifically, testing a middle-range theory of creativity, actualization, and empathy.

Michelle Benedict, R.N., B.S.N., is currently enrolled at the University of Michigan, pursuing a master's degree in the adult nurse practitioner program. She obtained her bachelor of science in nursing from Mercy College of Detroit in 1978. Since that time she has worked primarily in critical care and emergency nursing, holding positions in management, in education, and as a staff nurse. Presently, she is a staff nurse working in ambulatory surgery in a free-standing surgical center, where she is involved in developing patient education programs for patients undergoing surgery. Her incorporation and application of nursing theory into everyday nursing practices are inherent in whatever education or arena of nursing in which she is involved.

Charmaine Caron, M.Sc.N., is Assistant Executive Director, Nursing Services at Scarborough Grace Hospital in Scarborough, Ontario. Prior to accepting her current position, she was Director of Nursing Quality Assurance at Centenary Health Centre at Centenary.

Vivian Chan, M.Sc.N., was a Clinical Nurse Specialist in Medicine at Centenary Health Centre in Scarborough, Ontario, prior to accepting her current position as Director of Quality Management at Centenary.

Esther Coker, M.Sc.N., is a Clinical Education Specialist in Health Services for the Elderly at Chedoke-McMaster Hospitals in Hamilton, Ontario. She has lectured and coauthored articles on implementing King's systems framework at the bedside. Prior to moving to Hamilton, she was a Clinical Educator in Specialty Services at Centenary Health Centre.

Mary Molewyk Doornbos, B.S.N., M.S., Ph.D., is currently an Associate Professor of Nursing in the Hope-Calvin Department of Nursing at Calvin College in Grand Rapids, Michigan. In this capacity, she teaches the undergraduate theory and clinical courses in psychiatric nursing. She received her B.S.N. in 1980 and her M.S. in psychiatric-mental health nursing in 1983 from the University of Michigan. Her Ph.D. was granted from Wayne State University in 1993. Her chapter is based on her dissertation, *Family Health in the Families of the Young Chronically Mentally Ill*. She has presented papers and posters based on this research at local, regional, national, and international conferences. Her current research interests include further empirical testing of the middle-range theory of family health, particularly those modifications suggested by the initial data analysis.

Ginger W. Evans, M.S., M.S.N., R.N., C.S., is an Assistant Professor in the College of Nursing at the University of Tennessee at Knoxville. With 18 years' teaching experience, she currently coordinates the psychosocial long-term nursing course in the baccalaureate nursing program and the community mental health course in the nonnurse M.S.N. program. Clinically, she has been a nurse consultant providing mental status assessments and recommendations, group and individual counseling, and educational classes to a cardiac rehabilitation program. Currently, she is a consultant evaluating the use of psychoactive medications in the geriatric population. She received her master's in child and family studies and a master of science in nursing from the University of Tennessee at Knoxville and a B.S.N. from East Tennessee State University. Her research interests include teaching in the affective domain, empathy, and families caring for the chronically mentally ill.

J. Mary Fawcett, R.N., B.Sc.N., M.H.Sc., C.N.N.(c), is a graduate of the School of Nursing, Faculty of Health Sciences, McMaster University, Hamilton, Ontario. She has held positions in medical-surgical nursing as a staff nurse, nurse manager, and a supervisor. For the past 15 years, she has held a joint appointment as a Professor in the School of Nursing, Faculty of Health Sciences, McMaster University, and as a Clinical Nurse Specialist, Neurosciences, at Hamilton Civic Hospitals, General Division, Hamilton, Ontario. This position enables her to both teach and participate in the application of nursing theories at the bedside.

Jacqueline Fawcett, Ph.D., F.A.A.N., is a Professor at the University of Pennsylvania School of Nursing in Philadelphia. She is the author of four books dealing with nursing knowledge development: *Analysis and Evaluation of Conceptual Models of Nursing, Analysis and Evaluation of Nursing Theories, The Relationship of Theory and Research* (with Florence Downs), and *Family Theory Development in Nursing: State of the Science and Art* (with Ann Whall).

Thelma Fradley, B.Sc.N., now retired, was the Director of Specialty Services at Centenary Health Centre in Scarborough, Ontario, where she chaired the Nursing Practice Subcommittee of the Nursing Quality Assurance Committee during the categorization project.

Maureen A. Frey, Ph.D., is an Assistant Professor of Nursing at the University of Michigan School of Nursing. Her teaching and research interests are in nursing theory development, testing nursing theories, child/adolescent and family health, and chronic illness. She is also part of the clinical nursing faculty at the University of Michigan Medical Center, Department of Ambulatory Care, and sees children and families in the Diabetes Clinic. She received her M.S.N. and Ph.D. in nursing from Wayne State University, Detroit, Michigan.

Dorothy Froman, M.N., R.N., is currently Consultant, Professional Issues, for the Manitoba Association of Registered Nurses, Winnipeg, Manitoba, Canada. She obtained her B.N. from the University of Victoria, Victoria, British Columbia, her B.A. in cultural anthropology from the University of Winnipeg, Winnipeg, Manitoba, and her M.N. from the University of Manitoba, Winnipeg, Manitoba. Her interest in King began in 1981 when she coordinated the development of a 2-year diploma, registered nursing program curriculum based on King's theory. She continues to be an advocate of applying nursing theory in the clinical practice setting.

Kathleen M. Hanna, Ph.D., R.N., has had numerous years of experience in parent-child/adolescent nursing. Her clinical experience has included nursing of children and adolescents in acute care and ambulatory settings. Her educational background includes a M.S.N. (maternal-child) from the University of Nebraska Medical Center and a Ph.D. in nursing (parent-child) from the University of Pittsburgh. Her research interest is in the area of adolescents' health beliefs and behaviors.

Janet Harris, M.Sc.N., is Program Administrator, Neuro and Transplant, at the Toronto Hospital in Toronto, Ontario. Prior to accepting her position she was Director of Nursing at Centenary Health Centre.

Elizabeth F. Hobdell, Ph.D., R.N., C.N.R.N., is currently a Clinical Specialist in Child Neurology at St. Christopher's Hospital for Children in Philadelphia. She received her undergraduate education from Villanova University and did her master's and doctoral work at the University of Pennsylvania. She used King's framework for her dissertation research. Her special interests are in administration and psychosocial aspects of child and parent care. Her research interests include the effect of nursing care activities on intracranial pressure in children and the relationship between chronic sorrow and accuracy of perception of cognitive development in parents of children with neural tube defect.

Mary Lue Jolly, Ph.D., is an Associate Professor in the College of Nursing at the University of Tennessee at Knoxville. She coordinates the nursing administration concentration in the master's program and teaches health policy and management courses in the doctoral program at the University of Tennessee. Previously, she has been a staff nurse, head nurse, supervisor, and director of nursing service in hospitals in Ohio and Tennessee. She was also on the faculty at the University of Cincinnati College of Nursing and Health. She received her doctorate in education from the University of Kentucky, her master's with a major in administration of nursing services from Teachers College of Columbia University, New York, and a bachelor of arts with a major in chemistry from Edgecliff College, Cincinnati, Ohio. She earned her diploma in nursing at Mercy Hospital, Hamilton, Ohio. Her research interests are in organizational culture, systems testing, and the nurse-physician relationship in hospital practice.

Tomomi Kameoka, M.S.N., is a nurse at Shiga University Hospital, Shiga Perfecture, Japan. Her research interests are in theory development, testing King's theory, adult nursing, and basic nursing education. She received her M.S.N. from Chiba University.

Imogene M. King, R.N., Ed.D, F.A.A.N., graduated from a diploma school of nursing in 1945 and enrolled in a program at St. Louis University, where she completed a bachelor of science degree with a major in nursing and in education and a minor in philosophy and chemistry. For 12 years, she served as practitioner-teacher, during which time she completed a master of science degree in nursing and in administration at St. Louis University. She entered Teachers College, Columbia University, New York, in the fall of 1959 and completed a doctor of education degree in the spring of 1961. Her initial faculty position at Loyola University in Chicago included teaching and administration, during which time she developed and implemented a graduate program to prepare clinical specialists in adult nursing and teachers and administrators for associate degree nursing programs. This was the first master's program based on a nurse's conceptual framework (1968-1972). In her position as the nurse administrator at Ohio State University, Dr. M. Kaufman developed and implemented the first undergraduate curriculum based on her systems framework, a program deemed by faculty reports as very successful. She served as a Professor of Nursing at the University of South Florida, Tampa, Florida, teaching graduate students theory, research, curriculum, and adult nursing. During her 10 years in Florida, she served as a resource person and coteacher in the new doctoral program in nursing at the University of Miami. Currently, she is a Professor Emeritus, University of South Florida, Tampa, where she is a guest lecturer on her theory. She is also a consultant for several studies testing her theory. In addition, she is a resource person for several doctoral students developing theories from her systems framework. She has been invited as a consultant in hospitals where the nurses have selected her systems framework as the basis for their practice. Recent publications include "Quality of Life and Goal Attainment" (*Nursing Science Quarterly*, 1994). She is also coediting a monograph on the language of theory.

Joyce K. Laben, R.N., M.S.N., J.D., F.A.A.N., is a Professor of Psychiatric Nursing at Vanderbilt University, where she currently coordinates the graduate psychiatric mental health specialty. She has worked for many years with individuals who have mental health problems and who are charged with crimes. She developed the modern-day forensic mental health program for the state of Tennessee. She is a coauthor of two editions of a book on mental health law for nurses. She is a clinician with mental health services at the Vine Hill Community Clinic in Nashville, Tennessee, a nurse-run clinic.

Patricia R. Messmer, Ph.D., received a diploma in nursing from Presbyterian University Hospital and a B.S.N. from the University of Pittsburgh; an M.S.N. and an M.A. in rehabilitation counseling from Edinboro University of Pennsylvania, Edinboro, Pennsylvania; and a Ph.D. in higher education/educational administration from the University of Pittsburgh. Currently, she is Director of Nursing Research at Mount Sinai Medical Center in Miami Beach, Florida. Formerly, she was Director of Nursing Education and Research at Tampa General Hospital, Tampa, Florida. She holds adjunct faculty appointments at the University of Miami, Barry University, Florida International University, and the University of Florida. She held previous faculty appointments at Pennsylvania State University, University of Cincinnati, Villa Maria College/Gannon University, and Edinboro University of Pennsylvania. She is certified in ANA staff development and continuing education. She has published in the *Journal of Professional Nursing, Nurse Educator, Journal of Nursing Staff Development, Journal of Continuing Education in Nursing, Nursing Economics,* and *Florida Nurse.* She is on the editorial board of the *Journal of Nursing Staff Development* and has presented at a number of conferences. She is a member of ANA, NLN, NNSDO, Sigma Theta Tau, and the Southern Research Nursing Society and has worked extensively with King for the past 6 years.

Liselotte Rooke, Ph.D., R.N., R.N.T., teaches preresearch courses and master's courses, mainly in nursing conceptual models, nursing diagnostic reasoning, and the research process at the Malmo College of Health and Caring Sciences, Malmö, Sweden and at the Unit of Nursing Research, University of Lund (Sweden). She began her nursing career in 1964 (B.S.N.), and in 1970 she graduated as a nursing educator. From 1977 to 1991 she taught in the Program of Nursing Education, University of Lund. In 1990, she was awarded a Ph.D. from the Department of Educational Research, University of Lund; her thesis title was *Nursing and Theoretical Structures of Nursing: A Didactic Attempt to Develop the Practice of Nursing.* She has written textbooks in nursing conceptual models and nursing diagnosis. Her current research is among others focusing on the everyday knowledge of nurses. She is a member of the board of Nordic College of Caring

Sciences. Currently she is Nurse Research Director at the hospital of Helsingborg, Sweden.

Sandra S. Seidel, R.N.C.S., M.S.N., is a certified psychiatric clinical nurse specialist. She is currently an instructor for Vanderbilt School of Nursing and a clinician for the Vanderbilt Psychopharmachology Clinic in Nashville, Tennessee. She received her diploma in nursing from Rapid City Regional Hospital School of Nursing in Rapid City, South Dakota, in 1984; her B.S.N. from South Dakota State University in 1987; and her M.S.N. in psychiatric nursing from Vanderbilt University in Nashville, Tennessee in 1992. She has worked with all age levels in psychiatric nursing, both in the hospital setting and in industry.

Nancy C. Sharts-Hopko, Ph.D., R.N., is an Associate Professor at the Villanova University College of Nursing. Her nursing background is in the areas of maternal-infant, women's, and international health. Her research efforts over the past decade have focused on women's perceived well-being during various life transitions, such as menopause, hysterectomy, birth in a cross-cultural setting, migration, HIV infection, and cognition of breast cancer risk. Prior to her employment at Villanova University in 1986, she served as a consultant for the World Health Organization in Bangladesh and as a Presbyterian missionary in Tokyo. She earned her graduate degrees in nursing at New York University. She is a fellow of the American Academy of Nursing.

Christina L. Sieloff. B.S.N., M.S.N., received her degrees from Wayne State University in Detroit, Michigan. Currently, she is a doctoral candidate in nursing at the same university. Her dissertation will focus on the development, and initial reliability and validity testing, of an instrument designed to estimate the power of a nursing department within King's (1981) systems framework. Active in the American Nurses Association, she has also published five texts, two chapters, and several articles on subjects related to psychiatric nursing, nursing administration, and nursing theory.

Larry D. Sneed, R.N., M.S.N., C.S., is a graduate and former faculty member of the Vanderbilt University School of Nursing. His clinical interests include psychopharmacology, neurobiology and mental illness, and the treatment of Axis II diagnoses. He has served as a clinical consultant in program development with adolescents for facilities across the Southeast with particular emphasis on the development of programs for juvenile delinquent behavior and sexual offenders.

Dianne Tomarchio, A.D.N., is a staff nurse in the Coronary Care Unit at Centenary Health Centre. She has lectured on the unit's innovative approach to self-scheduling.

Valine M. Vaillancourt, R.N., B.Sc.N., B.A.M.Ed., is a graduate of the diploma nursing program at Humber College of Applied Arts and Technology in Toronto, Ontario. She received her B.Sc.N. and B.A. (psychology) from Laurentian University in Sudbury, Ontario. She completed her M.Ed. from Brock University, St. Catherine's, Ontario. Her thesis title was *Improving the Use of the Nursing Process: The Impact of a Charting Methodology Developed From King's Conceptual Framework on the Use of the Nursing Process.* She has held positions in psychiatry as a staff nurse and nurse manager. She has been a coordinator in a Home Health Care Program and has taught in the School of Nursing at Laurentian University. Currently, she is the Nursing Practice Clinician at the Hamilton Civic Hospitals, General Division, Hamilton, Ontario. This position enables her to facilitate the development of standards of patient care and policies and procedures that integrate theory into practice.

C. Annabelle Watson, R.N., B.Sc.N., is a graduate of a diploma nursing program from Victoria Hospital, London, Ontario. She received her B.Sc.N. from the University of Western Ontario in London, Ontario, and is currently working on her M.Sc.N. from D'Youville College in Buffalo, New York. She has held hospital positions as a staff nurse and clinical nursing educator and has taught for 12 years in college nursing faculty positions. Currently, she is the Nursing Practice Co-ordinator at the Hamilton Civic Hospitals, Henderson

General Division, Hamilton, Ontario. This position enables her to facilitate the integration of nursing theories into practice.

Ann L. Whall, Ph.D., F.A.A.N., is Professor in the School of Nursing at the University of Michigan—Ann Arbor. She is also Associate Director of the Geriatrics Center of the university. She has coauthored five textbooks dealing with the development of the theoretical knowledge base within nursing; two of these books received the American Nurses Association Book of the Year Award. She is also a Fellow in the Gerontology Society of America, and her work in this field concerns maintaining the functioning of late-stage dementia patients. Known also for her work in the development of family theory of nursing, she has been a guest lecturer at international conferences on this topic.

Mona Newsome Wicks, Ph.D., R.N., C.C.R.N., teaches medical-surgical nursing and critical care nursing at the University of Tennessee, Memphis College of Nursing, and is a clinical nurse at the Regional Medical Center (Critical Care Division). Prior to teaching, she was a staff nurse in pulmonary rehabilitation (for 3.5 years) and respiratory intensive care (for 6 years). She began her nursing career in 1978 as a graduate of Memphis State University receiving an A.D.N. In 1981, she was awarded a B.S.N. from Memphis State University; in 1987, an M.S.N. from the University of Tennessee; and in 1992, a Ph.D. from Wayne State University in Detroit, Michigan. She is a member of the Tennessee Nurses Association, the American Association of Critical Care Nurses, Sigma Theta Tau International, the Respiratory Nurses Society, and the Nightingale Society. She makes her home in Memphis with her husband Sammie and son Jamie.

Dorothy L. Wilt, B.S.N., M.S.N., was educated at Marquette University and the University of Tennessee. She is an Assistant Professor at the University of Tennessee at Knoxville. She has been a nurse educator for the past 17 years, with an intense interest in the phenomenon of teaching in the affective domain. She is also a nurse psychotherapist. She is a clinical member of the American Association of Marriage and Family Therapists and is a licensed family therapist in the state of Tennessee.

Cynthia Kelsey Winker holds a bachelor's degree in nursing from Baylor University in Texas and a master's degree in nursing administration from Northern Illinois University. She is currently a doctoral student at the University of Tennessee College of Nursing. She serves as Vice President of Marketing for AmSurg Corporation in Nashville, Tennessee. She has a broad range of experience in health care, including clinical nursing, nursing management, nursing education, and, most recently, health maintenance organizations operations management. She is a member of Sigma Theta Tau and a board member of the Tennessee Comprehensive Health Insurance Pool.

Made in the USA
Lexington, KY
27 October 2012